# THE COMPASSIONATE WARRIOR

# WEEKLY TOOLS

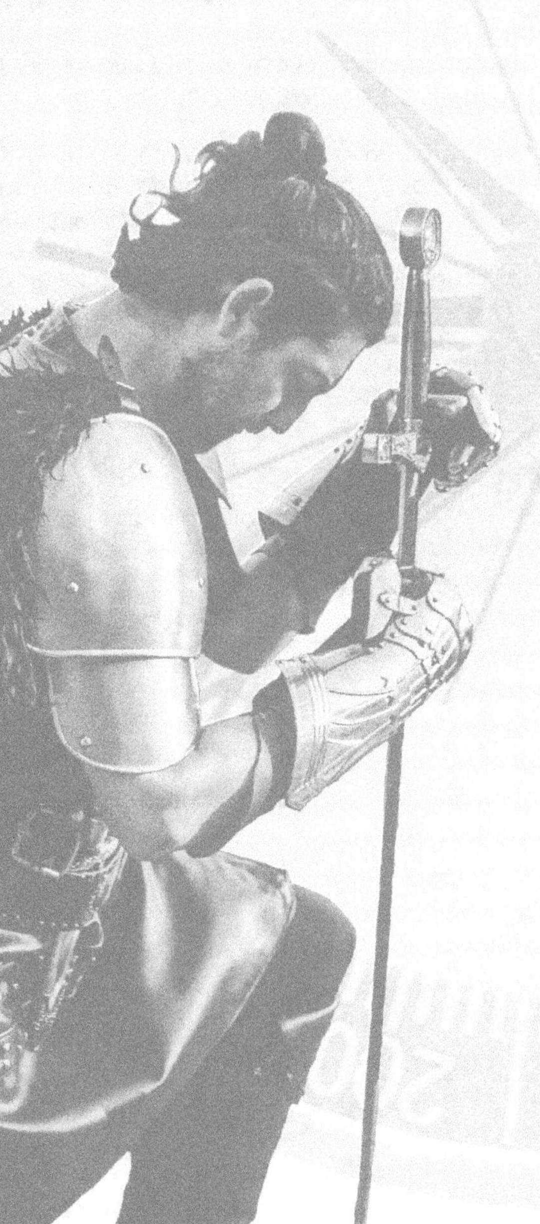

# The Compassionate Warrior Weekly Tools

Contributor:
Heather Kolb



Published by
Pure Desire Ministries International
886 NW Corporate Dr, Troutdale, OR 97060
www.puredesire.org | 503.489.0230

ISBN 978-1-943291-22-9



Content editing and copy editing by Heather Kolb

Typesetting by Emily Park and Elisabeth Windsor

Cover design and interior design by Elisabeth Windsor

# CONTENTS

# INTRODUCTION

## The Radical Journey Ahead

When we first entered the recovery journey, it was all about gaining and maintaining sobriety. We learned how our past pain and trauma contributed to our acting out behaviors. We discovered how our addictive behaviors had created chaos in our brain and we were given the tools we needed to renew our mind. We created healthy strategies to cope with and navigate the stresses of life. We've come a long way.

And now we stand on the cusp of our next-level healing journey. Our journey to become a Compassionate Warrior.

This journey is intended to take us deeper in our healing: deeper in our relationship with God, with the people we love, with our family and friends, and even with ourselves. This journey is holistic. It will address aspects of what we need to be healthy in several areas of our lives: physically, emotionally, relationally, sexually, and spiritually.

There's a lot that goes into our physical health: how much we exercise, our sleep habits, our relationship with food, and more. But learning how to practice self-care and creating a consistent plan will contribute to this holistic approach to healing.

Socially and culturally, men are not taught how to tend to their emotional health. They're not given permission or opportunity to express their feelings in a healthy way. And yet, if we're going to become a Compassionate Warrior, our emotional health needs to be developed. Our emotional health is directly tied to our relational health. Gaining strength in our emotional awareness will increase our ability to create healthy relationships.

As we continue to understand what it means to be sexually healthy, the more we recognize how our sexuality is tied to every area of our lives. We are sexual beings by God's design. Our sexuality is a core component of our identity. It's not something we can separate out or keep on the sidelines, but it needs to be an integrated part of who we are and who we are becoming. This is what it means to be holistically healthy.

In the same way, our spirituality is a deeply integrated part of who we are. It's not something that only shows up on Sunday at church. It's an active part of our healing, reflecting our relationship with God the Father, God the Son, and God the Holy Spirit. It is the foundation that gives us life and the guiding force that leads to lasting health and freedom.

This journey is no longer **only** about gaining sobriety and maintaining recovery; it **now includes** learning how to serve others. It's about being other-oriented. Our focus will be more on relationships and God's plan and purpose for our lives than on ourselves. It is about becoming the man God created us to be—becoming a Compassionate Warrior.

Everything in the *Weekly Tools* is for you and designed to move you to a deeper level of healing than you've experienced so far. It will expand your level of awareness and give you new tools to learn more about yourself and discover how you engage in relationships.

Although the *Weekly Tools* works in tandem with the *Workbook*, it is intended to help you develop new skills around your emotional health, how you communicate with others, the health of your thought life, self-care, and so much more. It's not just busywork or simply an extension of the *Workbook* lesson. It is focused on practical tools and assessments that will create a path to long term, holistic health.

Because of this approach, it will be best to do the *Weekly Tools* work separate from the *Workbook* work; at different times or different days throughout the week, so you can fully engage in this life-changing experience. And as with most experiences in life, the more we invest in it, the more we'll get out of it. Spending at least 30 minutes a day on your recovery work may be a minimum some weeks, but the investment in your recovery and healing is worth it!

The *Weekly Tools* contains some familiar tools as well as new tools that will be part of your weekly work. Here is a brief overview of the primary tools. Additional tools will be explained as they are introduced each week.

## Group Check-In

The Group Check-In contains two sections: "How did you do last week?" and "Where are you right now?"

**How did you do last week?** This section evaluates how we did last week, personally and in relationships.

We assess how we did on our commitment to change: a change in our thoughts, feelings, and behaviors that we chose to focus on throughout the week. Whether we chose to focus on an aspect of self-care (getting more exercise) or an issue identified on our FASTER Scale (repetitive negative thoughts), we made a commitment to intentionally change our behavior. This weekly practice keeps us moving forward in our healing.

We gauge our level of honesty, confessing whether we directly or indirectly lied to anyone. Learning to be honest with ourselves and others is an important part of our healing journey. It may not be our intention to lie, but even when we fail to tell the full truth about something—a lie of omission—it's a lie and hurts relationships. Raising awareness of our behaviors and intentionally practicing honesty is imperative to becoming a Compassionate Warrior.

We also identify what actions we're taking to improve our significant relationships.

**Where are you right now?** The one question in this section considers where we're at on the FASTER Scale for the week: how far down the FASTER Scale did we slide?

Complete the Group Check-In 24 hours before group.

## The FASTER Relapse Awareness Scale

If we want to change unwanted behaviors, we need to become more self-aware. Created by Michael Dye, the FASTER Relapse Awareness Scale (FASTER Scale) is designed to help identify patterns in our behaviors—patterns that lead to relapse.[1] These patterns reflect changes that are happening in us and around us: neurologically, psychologically, and socially.

When something stressful happens and we react suddenly or without much thought, we can end up relapsing and not really understand how we got there again. And yet, if we take the time to evaluate what was happening in our world in the days or weeks leading up to this relapse, it would become clear. We all experience thoughts, feelings, and behaviors that lead to our reactions. At the time, we are simply unaware.

Through the use of the FASTER Scale, we will become more aware of the thoughts, feelings, and behaviors that create the slippery slope toward relapse.

Each letter in the word "FASTER" represents a level on the scale: **F**orgetting priorities—**A**nxiety—**S**peeding up—**T**icked off—**E**xhausted—**R**elapse. Each level lists thoughts, feelings, attitudes, and actions that describe what someone is experiencing as they're descending toward relapse. Influenced by various factors— environmental stress, relationship issues, our physical and mental health—we find ourselves reacting to what is happening around us.

The FASTER Scale includes two parts: identification and evaluation.[2] Part one focuses on identification—within each step of the scale we will identify the thoughts, feelings, and behaviors we're experiencing throughout the week. We want to pay close attention to the thoughts, feelings, and behaviors that seem most powerful or show up with greater frequency throughout the week.

---

[1] Michael Dye, *The Genesis Process: For Change Groups, Book 1 and 2, Individual Workbook*, 4th ed. (Auburn: Michael Dye, 2012), 236.

[2] Michael Dye, *The Genesis Process*, 238.

Part two focuses on evaluation—using the most powerful or frequent thought, feeling, or behavior in each level, we will answer a set of questions. These questions will help us evaluate what's happening in our environment, contributing to where we are on the FASTER Scale. This raises awareness. Identifying and evaluating our thoughts, feelings, and behaviors enables us to create change.

One of the best things about the FASTER Scale is we don't have to work our way back up the scale. When we recognize where we are at—when we are sliding toward relapse—we simply step off and start doing the things that contribute to our restoration: accepting life on God's terms, with trust, grace, mercy, vulnerability, and gratitude.

This is a great tool for recognizing and changing behavior.

# Commitment to Change

Our Commitment to Change is often directly connected to the lowest level reached on the FASTER Scale, which is why it follows the FASTER Scale in the *Weekly Tools*.

**Let's plan for next week.** This section helps us plan ahead—what challenges are we facing and what is our new Commitment to Change for the coming week? What is our double bind—what lose-lose situation is driving a choice we have to make? How do we plan to maintain restoration and who will keep us accountable this next week?

As mentioned, a double bind is a lose-lose situation we face that will require a choice: the choice to stay the same or the choice to make a change. And both of these choices will cost us something. If we choose to stay the same, it often pulls us into isolation and leads to broken relationships. If we choose to change, even if it's difficult, it often leads to a closer relationship with God and others and contributes to lasting health.

Accountability is a huge part of this healing journey. Connecting with group members throughout the week will give us the support and encouragement we need to successfully complete this journey. Each week, we will call three group members, discuss how our week is going, and how we're doing with our Commitment to Change for the week.

During the week, especially if we're experiencing stress and recognize we're sliding toward relapse on the FASTER Scale, calling a group member can provide the encouragement we need to get back to restoration. This call is intentional. Our group is a lifeline—the men in our group are there for support when we need it.

When we have a plan in place—a plan centered in community and relationship with others—we are more likely to stay in restoration. As we embark on this Hero's Journey, this contributes to our lifelong healing.

**Complete the Commitment to Change before your next group meeting.**

# Stage Wrap Up

This study takes you through eight stages of the Hero's Journey. In many ways, this journey invites you on an adventure of exploration, discovery, and transformation—all of which is necessary for the life-changing experience of becoming a Compassionate Warrior.

As you complete each stage of this journey, you will find a Stage Wrap Up that includes three sections: 1) What Do You Think?, 2) Progress, Not Perfection, and 3) the Thoughts & Feelings Awareness Log.

**What Do You Think?** This section gives you the opportunity to journal about anything and everything. When you give yourself time to reflect on what you're learning, areas you're beginning to see change, and even what's taking up brain space, it brings healing to your mind and soul. It allows you to analyze how this journey is impacting you in both your challenges and successes.

**Progress, Not Perfection.** True and lasting change happens over time, one small change after another. Too often, when we become focused on the big change we're waiting to see happen, we miss out on seeing the small changes that are proof of our progress. This journey is not about perfection. It's about progress; all the steps we take and the changes that happen to transform us into the man God has called us to be.

This section will allow you to track the small changes that reflect the progress you're making: progress in your emotional health; progress in relationships; progress in self-care; progress in any area you're working on and investing in to create positive change in your life.

**Thoughts & Feelings Awareness Log.** This has happened to all of us: we experience an unexpected **event or situation**, which creates a tsunami of **thoughts and feelings** about the event or situation, motivating an **action or behavior**, resulting in the **outcome or circumstance** we find ourselves in. It's safe to say that our thoughts influence our feelings, our feelings influence our behaviors, and our behaviors influence our circumstances.

Many men have not been taught well or encouraged to develop their emotional health. And yet, men are emotional. Men have feelings. So denying this part of who they are can be damaging to them and their relationships.

Learning how our thoughts and feelings are connected and how they contribute to our behaviors is a huge part of this healing journey. Proactively attending to our thought life and increasing our emotional awareness will help us change our behaviors and make significant strides in our relationships.

**The Stage Wrap Up is for you: to assess what you're learning and how you're practically applying it to your healing journey.**

Lastly, each lesson should take a week to complete. However, there may be times when the discussion and/or content take two weeks to cover. So, additional weekly tools are included in the appendix for lessons that extend across two weeks.

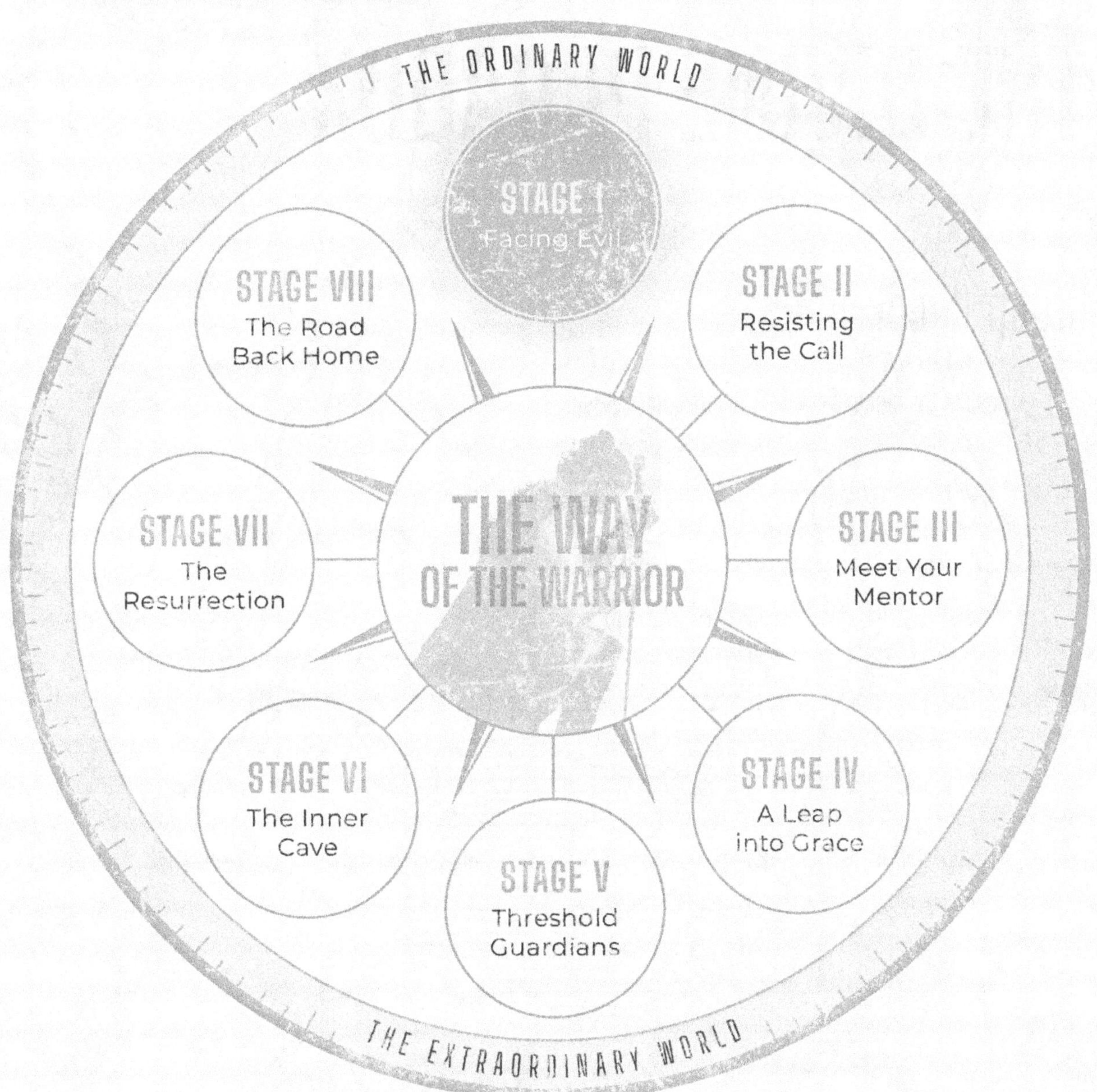


# STAGE I

## FACING EVIL

# CHAPTER 1
# THE DIVINE PARADOX

## Group Check-In

Complete the Group Check-In 24 hours before group.

### HOW DID YOU DO LAST WEEK?

Question 1 will be added next week.

02. Did you lie directly or indirectly to anyone? ______

03. What did you do to improve significant relationships with your wife, family, or friends? ______

### WHERE ARE YOU RIGHT NOW?

04. What is the lowest level you identify with on the FASTER Scale? ______

# Destructive Beliefs

Many of us develop destructive beliefs over time based on our life experiences. These destructive beliefs often stem from our interpretation of a situation and the thoughts and feelings we have based on the experience. For example: as a child, if we experienced a situation that was painful and traumatic, our brain would capture and store the thoughts and feelings created during the experience. This is how our brain, specifically the limbic system, was designed to keep us safe and help us survive potentially harmful and life-threatening situations.

However, our ability to understand and process an experience is based on several factors that were present at the time of the event: age, family dynamics, life stressors such as moving, parents divorcing, death of a family member, and more. To some degree, this may lead to misperceptions or cognitive distortions that fuel our destructive beliefs.

## COMMON MISPERCEPTIONS INCLUDE:[3]

**Rationalization:** creating excuses for the attitudes and actions of yourself and others that led to poor choices or an unhealthy outcome. This is a defense mechanism used to minimize emotional pain.

**Overgeneralization:** taking the basis of one or two personal experiences and applying it as an overall general pattern. For example, if a man's wife cheats on him, he may develop an overgeneralization that "all women are unfaithful."

**All-or-nothing thinking:** a perspective based on only two extremes: black or white; good or bad; positive or negative. Not leaving room for the gray and the potential for all the other variables that exist between the extremes.

**Discounting the positive:** rejecting positive experiences in an attempt to maintain a negative self-perception. For example, a man is given a positive job review, but attributes it to "my boss gives everyone a positive review."

**Fortune telling:** anticipating something bad is going to happen and predicting a negative outcome based on previous experiences. This type of thinking is caught up in "What if..." scenarios.

**Mind reading:** a belief that we know what someone else is thinking, often with a strong negative interpretation. This usually results in communication problems.

---

[3] Jeff Riggenbach, *The CBT Toolbox: A Workbook for Clients and Clinicians* (Eau Claire: Premier Publishing and Media, 2013), 9-10.

**Should statements:** placing unrealistic expectations on yourself or others, which results in feelings of anger, guilt, or disappointment. Common words or phrases include, "I must...," "I need to...," I ought to..."

**Emotional reasoning:** presuming that your negative feelings accurately reflect reality. Contributes to the false interpretation of *Because I feel it, it must be true*.

**Magnification:** exaggerating the importance of something and blowing it way out of proportion. This often includes catastrophizing the meaning or perceived outcome of a situation or event.

**Personalization:** seeing yourself as the cause of a negative situation, when you had nothing to do with it. Making something about you when it's not, resulting in hurt feelings.

**Which of these misperceptions tend to show up most in your thought processes and fuel your destructive beliefs?** A couple examples are given to get you started.

| MISPERCEPTION | DESTRUCTIVE BELIEF |
|---|---|
| All-or-nothing thinking | If I'm not successful at everything I do, I'm a failure and always will be. |
| Mind reading | Even when my wife smiles at me, I know she's faking. She thinks I'm the loser who ruined her life. |
| | |
| | |
| | |
| | |

Understanding how our misconceptions fuel our destructive beliefs can be a powerful tool when it comes to changing how this affects our relationships.

Think of a situation with your wife (or a close relationship, if you're not married) in which your misperception contributed to a negative outcome. Explain.

If this situation were to happen again, what would you do differently to bring about a more positive outcome?

What misconception and/or destructive belief do you want to work to dismantle throughout this healing journey?

The greatest challenge we face throughout this journey is change: being willing to learn and grow as we pursue the lifelong healing God has for our lives. The greatest reward we receive throughout this journey is change: becoming the Compassionate Warrior God created us to be.

# FASTER Scale[4]

Circle the behaviors on the FASTER Scale that you identify with in each section.
Identify the most powerful behavior in each section and write it next to the corresponding heading.
Answer the following three questions based on your most powerful or frequent behavior.

01. How does it affect me? How do I feel in the moment?
02. How does it affect the important people in my life?
03. Why do I do this? What is the benefit for me?[5]

## RESTORATION ____________________

*(Accepting life on God's terms, with trust, grace, mercy, vulnerability and gratitude.)* No current secrets; working to resolve problems; identifying fears and feelings; keeping commitments to meetings, prayer, family, church, people, goals, and self; being open and honest, making eye contact; increasing in relationships with God and others; true accountability.

01. ____________________
02. ____________________
03. ____________________

## FORGETTING PRIORITIES ____________________

*(Start believing the present circumstances and moving away from trusting God. Denial; flight; a change in what's important; how you spend your time, energy, and thoughts.)* Secrets; less time/energy for God, meetings, church; avoiding support and accountability people; superficial conversations; sarcasm; isolating; changes in goals; obsessed with relationships; breaking promises and commitments; neglecting family; preoccupation with material things, TV, computers, entertainment; procrastination; lying; overconfidence; bored; hiding money; image management; seeking to control situations and other people.

01. ____________________
02. ____________________
03. ____________________

---

[4] Michael Dye, *The Genesis Process: For Change Groups, Book 1 and 2, Individual Workbook*, 4th ed. (Auburn: Michael Dye, 2012), 236.

[5] For question 3, keep in mind: everything we do, we do because it meets a legitimate need. Even when we engage in unhealthy or destructive behaviors, we're doing it because it's meeting a need. One of the most rewarding aspects of our healing comes from figuring out our legitimate needs and finding healthy ways to meet these needs.

## ANXIETY

*(Consumed by negative thoughts and undefined fear; getting energy from emotions.)* Worry, using profanity, being fearful; being resentful; replaying old, negative thoughts; perfectionism; judging other's motives; making goals and lists that you can't complete; mind reading; fantasy, codependent, rescuing; sleep problems, trouble concentrating, seeking/creating drama; gossip; using over-the-counter medication for pain, sleep or weight control; flirting.

01. ______

02. ______

03. ______

## SPEEDING UP

*(Trying to outrun the anxiety which is usually the first sign of depression.)* Super busy and always in a hurry (finding good reason to justify the work); workaholic; can't relax; avoiding slowing down; feeling driven; can't turn off thoughts; skipping meals; binge eating (usually at night); overspending; can't identify own feelings/needs; repetitive negative thoughts; irritable; dramatic mood swings; too much caffeine; over exercising; nervousness; difficulty being alone and/or with people; difficulty listening to others; making excuses for having to "do it all."

01. ______

02. ______

03. ______

## TICKED OFF

*(Getting adrenaline high on anger and aggression.)* Procrastination causing crisis in money, work, and relationships; increased sarcasm; black and white (all or nothing) thinking; feeling alone; nobody understands; overreacting, road rage; constant resentments; pushing others away; increasing isolation; blaming; arguing; irrational thinking; can't take criticism; defensive; people avoiding you; needing to be right; digestive problems; headaches; obsessive (stuck) thoughts; can't forgive; feeling superior; using intimidation.

01. ____________________

02. ____________________

03. ____________________

## EXHAUSTED

*(Loss of physical and emotional energy; coming off the adrenaline high, and the onset of depression.)* Depressed; panicked; confused; hopelessness; sleeping too much or too little; can't cope; overwhelmed; crying for "no reason"; can't think; forgetful; pessimistic; helpless; tired; numb; wanting to run; constant cravings for old coping behaviors; thinking of using sex, drugs, or alcohol; seeking old unhealthy people and places; really isolating; people angry with you; self abuse; suicidal thoughts; spontaneous crying; no goals; survival mode; not returning phone calls; missing work; irritability; no appetite.

01. ____________________

02. ____________________

03. ____________________

## RELAPSE

*(Returning to the place you swore you would never go again. Coping with life on your terms. You sitting in the driver's seat instead of God.)* Giving up and giving in; out of control; lost in your addiction; lying to yourself and others; feeling you just can't manage without your coping behaviors, at least for now. The result is the reinforcement of shame, guilt and condemnation; and feelings of abandonment and being alone.

01. ____________________

02. ____________________

03. ____________________

# Commitment To Change

Complete the Commitment to Change prior to your next group meeting.

Keep in mind, your Commitment to Change is often directly connected to the lowest level reached on the FASTER Scale. Healing happens best when we are fully aware of the challenges we face and take proactive steps to create change.

## LET'S PLAN FOR NEXT WEEK

Commitment to change: what area do you need to change or what challenge are you facing this week?

- Double bind: what will it cost you if you change? If you don't change?
- How does this potential for change make you feel?
- What is your plan to maintain restoration regarding these changes?

Who will you share your commitment with this week?

What are the details of your accountability? What questions should they ask you?

BE PREPARED TO SHARE YOUR ANSWERS IN THIS CHAPTER WITH THE GUYS IN YOUR GROUP.

# CHAPTER 2
# TAKING UP THE SWORD

## Group Check-In

Complete the Group Check-In 24 hours before group.

### HOW DID YOU DO LAST WEEK?

01. How did you do on your Commitment to Change? ____________________

02. Did you lie directly or indirectly to anyone? ____________________

03. What did you do to improve significant relationships with your wife, family, or friends? ____________________

### WHERE ARE YOU RIGHT NOW?

04. What is the lowest level you identify with on the FASTER Scale? ____________________

# Developing Emotional Health

Life is all about transitions and how we handle transitions will have a lot to do with the depth and strength of character we develop.

This is especially true when it comes to our emotional health. If we are going to become a Compassionate Warrior who is sensitive to the needs of others, we need to learn how to express our feelings in a healthy way. This requires awareness and balance.

Many of us grew up believing this unspoken secret: a real man doesn't show his emotions but becomes an expert at suppressing his emotions. Even if no one actually said this out loud to us, it was implied through countless experiences. As we venture further into our healing journey, learning the importance of emotional regulation can be challenging and confusing.

Consider these situations and the emotional component in each:

## SITUATION #1:

Your son is playing outside and falls. The fall breaks his arm and, although you immediately feel a host of emotions, you need to suppress your feelings in order to act quickly and get your son to the emergency room. Several hours later, after your son is out of surgery and resting in recovery, you become overwhelmed with emotion. At last, you're able to release all the emotions you've been feeling but couldn't express until now.

## SITUATION #2:

You're at a sporting event with friends. Your favorite team is playing their biggest rival. The stands are packed and the emotions are high. Your team is behind and the refs have made a few poor calls. In your frustration, and because the environment allows for it, you have no problem yelling your disapproval at the refs or yelling to encourage your team when they make a great play. You are very aware of your emotions and freely express what you're feeling when you're feeling it.

## SITUATION #3:

You have a project deadline and have to work late. You communicate this to your wife and tell her when you'll be home. In order to focus on the project, you put your phone on silent. When you get home, your wife is angry and crying. She explains that she tried to call you and you didn't answer your phone. She immediately felt triggered by the possibility that you're acting out again. You say you're sorry, but suppress your other feelings because expressing them might sound like making excuses, which has only made things worse in the past.

Developing emotional health starts with awareness and is a process of recognizing how our thoughts, feelings, and actions are connected.[6] We often hear statements like this: "I felt like she was going to be mad no matter what I did. It was a lose-lose situation for sure!" This is not a feeling, but a perfect example of a thought. **Thoughts are often expressed in a full sentence. Feelings are often expressed in one word:** I felt sad, mad, happy, excited, overwhelmed, fortunate, grateful.

**The key to developing emotional health is practice. So consider again the previous situations and answer the following questions.**

## SITUATION #1:

What do you think are the benefits of suppressing and/or expressing emotion in this situation?

**What thoughts and feelings do you think this dad is experiencing?** (Thoughts are expressed in a full sentence; feelings are expressed in one word.)

**Thoughts:** ____________________

**Feelings:** ____________________

[6] Jeff Riggenbach, *The CBT Toolbox: A Workbook for Clients and Clinicians* (Eau Claire: Premier Publishing and Media, 2013), 3.

## SITUATION #2:

What do you think are the benefits of suppressing and/or expressing emotion in this situation?

______________________________________________

______________________________________________

______________________________________________

______________________________________________

**What thoughts and feelings do you think this guy is experiencing?** (Thoughts are expressed in a full sentence; feelings are expressed in one word.)

**Thoughts:** ______________________________________________

______________________________________________

**Feelings:** ______________________________________________

## SITUATION #3:

What do you think are the benefits of suppressing and/or expressing emotion in this situation?

______________________________________________

______________________________________________

______________________________________________

______________________________________________

**What thoughts and feelings do you think this husband is experiencing?** (Thoughts are expressed in a full sentence; feelings are expressed in one word.)

**Thoughts:** ______________________________________________

______________________________________________

**Feelings:** ______________________________________________

Becoming more emotionally aware will equip us to handle life's transitions with a greater understanding of who we are and create in us a sensitivity toward the needs of others.

# FASTER Scale

Circle the behaviors on the FASTER Scale that you identify with in each section.
Identify the most powerful behavior in each section and write it next to the corresponding heading.
Answer the following three questions based on your most powerful or frequent behavior.

01. How does it affect me? How do I feel in the moment?
02. How does it affect the important people in my life?
03. Why do I do this? What is the benefit for me?

## RESTORATION ______________________________

*(Accepting life on God's terms, with trust, grace, mercy, vulnerability and gratitude.)* No current secrets; working to resolve problems; identifying fears and feelings; keeping commitments to meetings, prayer, family, church, people, goals, and self; being open and honest, making eye contact; increasing in relationships with God and others; true accountability.

01. ______________________________
02. ______________________________
03. ______________________________

## FORGETTING PRIORITIES ______________________________

*(Start believing the present circumstances and moving away from trusting God. Denial; flight; a change in what's important; how you spend your time, energy, and thoughts.)* Secrets; less time/energy for God, meetings, church; avoiding support and accountability people; superficial conversations; sarcasm; isolating; changes in goals; obsessed with relationships; breaking promises and commitments; neglecting family; preoccupation with material things, TV, computers, entertainment; procrastination; lying; overconfidence; bored; hiding money; image management; seeking to control situations and other people.

01. ______________________________
______________________________
02. ______________________________
______________________________
03. ______________________________
______________________________

## ANXIETY

*(Consumed by negative thoughts and undefined fear; getting energy from emotions.)* Worry, using profanity, being fearful; being resentful; replaying old, negative thoughts; perfectionism; judging other's motives; making goals and lists that you can't complete; mind reading; fantasy, codependent, rescuing; sleep problems, trouble concentrating, seeking/creating drama; gossip; using over-the-counter medication for pain, sleep or weight control; flirting.

01. ______

02. ______

03. ______

## SPEEDING UP

*(Trying to outrun the anxiety which is usually the first sign of depression.)* Super busy and always in a hurry (finding good reason to justify the work); workaholic; can't relax; avoiding slowing down; feeling driven; can't turn off thoughts; skipping meals; binge eating (usually at night); overspending; can't identify own feelings/needs; repetitive negative thoughts; irritable; dramatic mood swings; too much caffeine; over exercising; nervousness; difficulty being alone and/or with people; difficulty listening to others; making excuses for having to "do it all."

01. ______

02. ______

03. ______

## TICKED OFF

*(Getting adrenaline high on anger and aggression.)* Procrastination causing crisis in money, work, and relationships; increased sarcasm; black and white (all or nothing) thinking; feeling alone; nobody understands; overreacting, road rage; constant resentments; pushing others away; increasing isolation; blaming; arguing; irrational thinking; can't take criticism; defensive; people avoiding you; needing to be right; digestive problems; headaches; obsessive (stuck) thoughts; can't forgive; feeling superior; using intimidation.

01. ______________________________________________

______________________________________________

02. ______________________________________________

______________________________________________

03. ______________________________________________

______________________________________________

## EXHAUSTED ______________________________________________

*(Loss of physical and emotional energy; coming off the adrenaline high, and the onset of depression.)* Depressed; panicked; confused; hopelessness; sleeping too much or too little; can't cope; overwhelmed; crying for "no reason"; can't think; forgetful; pessimistic; helpless; tired; numb; wanting to run; constant cravings for old coping behaviors; thinking of using sex, drugs, or alcohol; seeking old unhealthy people and places; really isolating; people angry with you; self abuse; suicidal thoughts; spontaneous crying; no goals; survival mode; not returning phone calls; missing work; irritability; no appetite.

01. ______________________________________________

______________________________________________

02. ______________________________________________

______________________________________________

03. ______________________________________________

______________________________________________

## RELAPSE ______________________________________________

*(Returning to the place you swore you would never go again. Coping with life on your terms. You sitting in the driver's seat instead of God.)* Giving up and giving in; out of control; lost in your addiction; lying to yourself and others; feeling you just can't manage without your coping behaviors, at least for now. The result is the reinforcement of shame, guilt and condemnation; and feelings of abandonment and being alone.

01. ______________________________________________

______________________________________________

02. ______________________________________________

______________________________________________

03. ______________________________________________

______________________________________________

# Commitment To Change

Complete the Commitment to Change prior to your next group meeting.

Keep in mind, your Commitment to Change is often directly connected to the lowest level reached on the FASTER Scale. Healing happens best when we are fully aware of the challenges we face and take proactive steps to create change.

## LET'S PLAN FOR NEXT WEEK

### Commitment to change: what area do you need to change or what challenge are you facing this week?

- Double bind: what will it cost you if you change? If you don't change?
- How does this potential for change make you feel?
- What is your plan to maintain restoration regarding these changes?

### Who will you share your commitment with this week?

### What are the details of your accountability? What questions should they ask you?

### BE PREPARED TO SHARE YOUR ANSWERS IN THIS CHAPTER WITH THE GUYS IN YOUR GROUP.

CHAPTER 3

# THE BIBLICAL WARRIOR

## Group Check-In

Complete the Group Check-In 24 hours before group.

### HOW DID YOU DO LAST WEEK?

01. How did you do on your Commitment to Change? ______________________

______________________________________________

______________________________________________

______________________________________________

02. Did you lie directly or indirectly to anyone? ______________________

______________________________________________

______________________________________________

______________________________________________

03. What did you do to improve significant relationships with your wife, family, or friends? ______________________

______________________________________________

______________________________________________

______________________________________________

### WHERE ARE YOU RIGHT NOW?

04. What is the lowest level you identify with on the FASTER Scale? __________

______________________________________________

______________________________________________

______________________________________________

# Holistic Health

The more we invest in this healing journey, the more we come to understand this truth: it's not only about becoming sexually healthy, it's about becoming holistically healthy. This approach considers the multidimensional health and healing of a person's life: physically, emotionally, relationally, sexually, and spiritually.

Use the following space to begin creating a holistic health plan.[7]

**Be specific about the positive and/or healthy behaviors you need to put in place on a daily or weekly basis that will support you on your healing journey. For each behavior you list, circle whether the need is daily or weekly.**

In order to be **physically** healthy, I need:

- ______________________________ daily/weekly
- ______________________________ daily/weekly
- ______________________________ daily/weekly
- ______________________________ daily/weekly
- ______________________________ daily/weekly
- ______________________________ daily/weekly
- ______________________________ daily/weekly
- ______________________________ daily/weekly

In order to be **emotionally** healthy, I need:

- ______________________________ daily/weekly
- ______________________________ daily/weekly
- ______________________________ daily/weekly
- ______________________________ daily/weekly
- ______________________________ daily/weekly
- ______________________________ daily/weekly
- ______________________________ daily/weekly
- ______________________________ daily/weekly

---

[7] Triangle SAA (2017). Spring Step Retreat. Track 1, Step 1. 51.

In order to be **relationally** healthy, I need:

- ____________________ daily/weekly
- ____________________ daily/weekly
- ____________________ daily/weekly
- ____________________ daily/weekly
- ____________________ daily/weekly
- ____________________ daily/weekly
- ____________________ daily/weekly

In order to be **sexually** healthy, I need:

- ____________________ daily/weekly
- ____________________ daily/weekly
- ____________________ daily/weekly
- ____________________ daily/weekly
- ____________________ daily/weekly
- ____________________ daily/weekly
- ____________________ daily/weekly

In order to be **spiritually** healthy, I need:

- ____________________ daily/weekly
- ____________________ daily/weekly
- ____________________ daily/weekly
- ____________________ daily/weekly
- ____________________ daily/weekly
- ____________________ daily/weekly
- ____________________ daily/weekly

Don't worry about filling in all the blanks. As you become more aware of what you need to be holistically healthy, come back to this exercise and fill it in. Also, consider adding some of these items on this list to your Three Circles/Relapse Prevention Tool. This is part of the process of learning how to practically walk out our healing.

# FASTER Scale

Circle the behaviors on the FASTER Scale that you identify with in each section.
Identify the most powerful behavior in each section and write it next to the corresponding heading.
Answer the following three questions based on your most powerful or frequent behavior.

01. How does it affect me? How do I feel in the moment?
02. How does it affect the important people in my life?
03. Why do I do this? What is the benefit for me?

## RESTORATION ____________________

*(Accepting life on God's terms, with trust, grace, mercy, vulnerability and gratitude.)* No current secrets; working to resolve problems; identifying fears and feelings; keeping commitments to meetings, prayer, family, church, people, goals, and self; being open and honest, making eye contact; increasing in relationships with God and others; true accountability.

01. ____________________
02. ____________________
03. ____________________

## FORGETTING PRIORITIES ____________________

*(Start believing the present circumstances and moving away from trusting God. Denial; flight; a change in what's important; how you spend your time, energy, and thoughts.)* Secrets; less time/energy for God, meetings, church; avoiding support and accountability people; superficial conversations; sarcasm; isolating; changes in goals; obsessed with relationships; breaking promises and commitments; neglecting family; preoccupation with material things, TV, computers, entertainment; procrastination; lying; overconfidence; bored; hiding money; image management; seeking to control situations and other people.

01. ____________________
____________________
02. ____________________
____________________
03. ____________________
____________________

## ANXIETY

*(Consumed by negative thoughts and undefined fear; getting energy from emotions.)* Worry, using profanity, being fearful; being resentful; replaying old, negative thoughts; perfectionism; judging other's motives; making goals and lists that you can't complete; mind reading; fantasy, codependent, rescuing; sleep problems, trouble concentrating, seeking/creating drama; gossip; using over-the-counter medication for pain, sleep or weight control; flirting.

01. ______________________________

02. ______________________________

03. ______________________________

## SPEEDING UP

*(Trying to outrun the anxiety which is usually the first sign of depression.)* Super busy and always in a hurry (finding good reason to justify the work); workaholic; can't relax; avoiding slowing down; feeling driven; can't turn off thoughts; skipping meals; binge eating (usually at night); overspending; can't identify own feelings/needs; repetitive negative thoughts; irritable; dramatic mood swings; too much caffeine; over exercising; nervousness; difficulty being alone and/or with people; difficulty listening to others; making excuses for having to "do it all."

01. ______________________________

02. ______________________________

03. ______________________________

## TICKED OFF

*(Getting adrenaline high on anger and aggression.)* Procrastination causing crisis in money, work, and relationships; increased sarcasm; black and white (all or nothing) thinking; feeling alone; nobody understands; overreacting, road rage; constant resentments; pushing others away; increasing isolation; blaming; arguing; irrational thinking; can't take criticism; defensive; people avoiding you; needing to be right; digestive problems; headaches; obsessive (stuck) thoughts; can't forgive; feeling superior; using intimidation.

01. ______________________________________________

______________________________________________

02. ______________________________________________

______________________________________________

03. ______________________________________________

______________________________________________

## EXHAUSTED

*(Loss of physical and emotional energy; coming off the adrenaline high, and the onset of depression.)* Depressed; panicked; confused; hopelessness; sleeping too much or too little; can't cope; overwhelmed; crying for "no reason"; can't think; forgetful; pessimistic; helpless; tired; numb; wanting to run; constant cravings for old coping behaviors; thinking of using sex, drugs, or alcohol; seeking old unhealthy people and places; really isolating; people angry with you; self abuse; suicidal thoughts; spontaneous crying; no goals; survival mode; not returning phone calls; missing work; irritability; no appetite.

01. ______________________________________________

______________________________________________

02. ______________________________________________

______________________________________________

03. ______________________________________________

______________________________________________

## RELAPSE

*(Returning to the place you swore you would never go again. Coping with life on your terms. You sitting in the driver's seat instead of God.)* Giving up and giving in; out of control; lost in your addiction; lying to yourself and others; feeling you just can't manage without your coping behaviors, at least for now. The result is the reinforcement of shame, guilt and condemnation; and feelings of abandonment and being alone.

01. ______________________________________________

______________________________________________

02. ______________________________________________

______________________________________________

03. ______________________________________________

______________________________________________

# Commitment To Change

Complete the Commitment to Change prior to your next group meeting.

Keep in mind, your Commitment to Change is often directly connected to the lowest level reached on the FASTER Scale. Healing happens best when we are fully aware of the challenges we face and take proactive steps to create change.

## LET'S PLAN FOR NEXT WEEK

Commitment to change: what area do you need to change or what challenge are you facing this week?

- Double bind: what will it cost you if you change? If you don't change?
- How does this potential for change make you feel?
- What is your plan to maintain restoration regarding these changes?

Who will you share your commitment with this week?

What are the details of your accountability? What questions should they ask you?

BE PREPARED TO SHARE YOUR ANSWERS IN THIS CHAPTER WITH THE GUYS IN YOUR GROUP.

# STAGE I
# WRAP UP

## What do you think?

Writing by hand does amazing things for your brain. Research suggests writing by hand creates event-related synchrony in several areas of the brain, which contributes to encoding and remembering new information.[8] This is one of the best ways to retain and apply the new things we're learning. It also facilitates getting our thoughts out of our head—putting them on paper—where we can see them and they become real.

For some, this might be an easy task because journaling is already part of your routine. For others, this might feel like torture because you've never found journaling helpful in the past. Regardless of where you might fall between these two extremes, handwriting does promote a healthy brain and contributes to healing in many ways.

Take some time to write about what you've learned so far in Stage I of this Hero's Journey.

[8] Eva Ose Askvik, F. R. van der Weel, & Audrey L. H. van der Meer, The Importance of Cursive Handwriting Over Typewriting for Learning in the Classroom: A High-Density EEG Study of 12-Year-Old Children and Young Adults, *Frontiers in Psychology*, 11:1810, July 28, 2020, https://doi.org/10.3389/fpsyg.2020.01810.

# Progress, Not Perfection[9]

Perfectionism and addictive behaviors seem to run in the same circles. Many men who have struggled with compulsive sexual behaviors also struggle with perfectionism. But as we become healthy, we recognize that **this journey is about progress, not perfection.**

Since lifelong change happens in small increments, we can become impatient and lose sight of the progress we're actually making. Tracking even the smallest progress can be encouraging and help us maintain forward motion toward our goals and overall healing.

### Use the following tables to note areas where you're making day-to-day progress.

It is common for us to have several areas we're working on at the same time, so there are no wrong answers here. The purpose of this is to raise awareness of our small successes and keep our momentum going. Here are a couple examples to get you started.

*Examples:*

| ISSUE | PERFECTION | WHERE I STARTED | PROGRESS |
|---|---|---|---|
| *Lack of exercise* | *Exercise for 2 hours every day* | *Getting no exercise at all* | *Exercising for 45 minutes 4 times a week* |

### What can you do this week to make progress toward your goal?

*Find an additional day to exercise or keep my current days and add another 15 minutes to my time.*

| ISSUE | PERFECTION | WHERE I STARTED | PROGRESS |
|---|---|---|---|
| *I need to make time for date nights with my wife* | *A date night every week* | *A date night every few months* | *We've had a date night every other week for the past two months* |

[9] Jeff Riggenbach, *The CBT Toolbox: A Workbook for Clients and Clinicians* (Eau Claire: Premier Publishing and Media, 2013), 39-40.

What can you do this week to make progress toward your goal?

*Talk with my wife about scheduling a third date night this month.*

Now it's your turn. How are you making progress in your goals and overall healing?

| ISSUE | PERFECTION | WHERE I STARTED | PROGRESS |
| --- | --- | --- | --- |
| | | | |

What can you do this week to make progress toward your goal?

| ISSUE | PERFECTION | WHERE I STARTED | PROGRESS |
| --- | --- | --- | --- |
| | | | |

What can you do this week to make progress toward your goal?

| ISSUE | PERFECTION | WHERE I STARTED | PROGRESS |
| --- | --- | --- | --- |
| | | | |

What can you do this week to make progress toward your goal?

# Thoughts & Feelings Awareness Log[10]

Our thoughts and feelings influence our behaviors. Raising awareness to this connection takes time and practice. Use the following table to analyze how your thoughts and feelings are affecting your behaviors at this stage of your journey. The Feeling Wheel[11] is included to help identify what you're feeling. A couple examples are given to get you started. (Remember from Chapter 2: feelings are one word, thoughts are a full sentence.)

| I FELT… | …BECAUSE I THOUGHT… |
|---|---|
| *Angry, worthless, insignificant* | *I was going to be passed over, again, for the promotion.* |
| *Disrespected, invisible, rejected* | *When my family planned a weekend away without asking for my thoughts and opinions about it.* |
| | |
| | |
| | |

[10] Jeff Riggenbach, *The CBT Toolbox: A Workbook for Clients and Clinicians* (Eau Claire: Premier Publishing and Media, 2013), 17.

[11] Gloria Willcox, "The Feeling Wheel: A Tool for Expanding Awareness of Emotions and Increasing Spontaneity and Intimacy," *Transactional Analysis Journal*, Vol. 12, No. 4, October 1982.

# The Feeling Wheel[12]

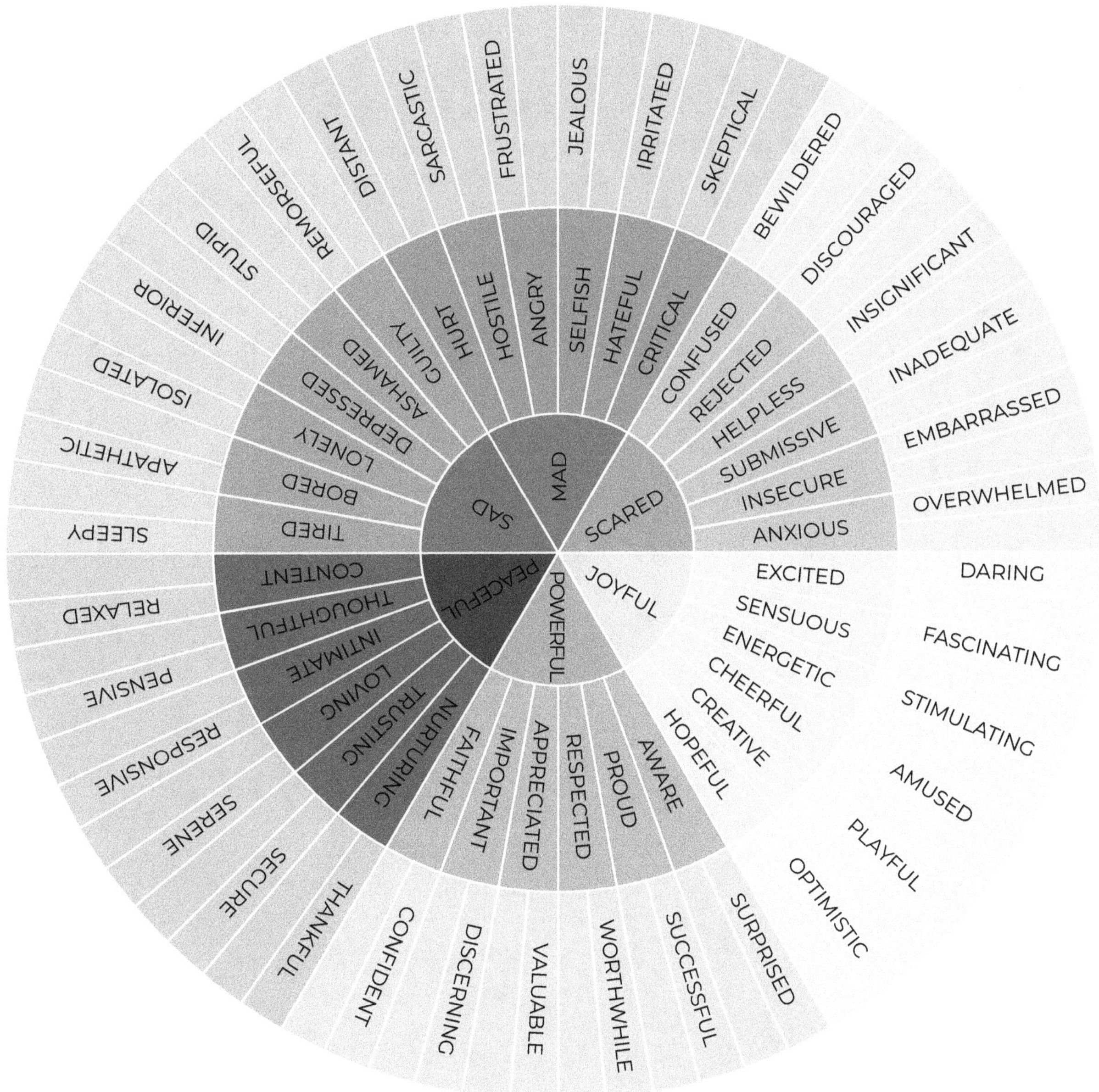


The journaling and tools in this wrap up are for you, so you can evaluate what you're learning and keep track of the progress you're making. You don't have to share any of this with the guys in your group, but can if you want to.

---

[12] Gloria Willcox, "The Feeling Wheel: A Tool for Expanding Awareness of Emotions and Increasing Spontaneity and Intimacy," *Transactional Analysis Journal*, Vol. 12, No. 4, October 1982.

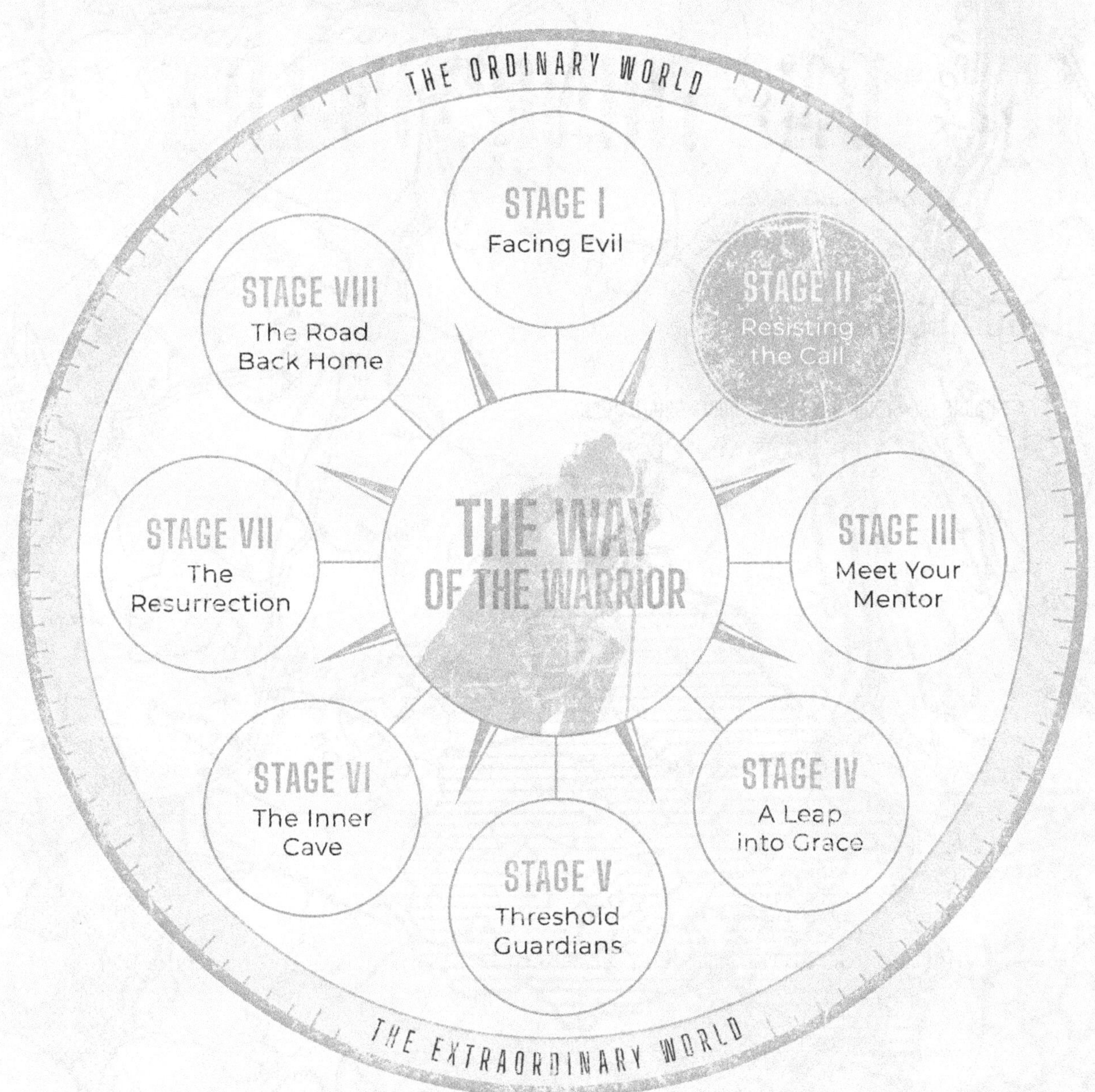


# STAGE II

## RESISTING THE CALL

CHAPTER 4

# THE "ONE THING" IN LIFE

## Group Check-In

Complete the Group Check-In 24 hours before group.

### HOW DID YOU DO LAST WEEK?

01. How did you do on your Commitment to Change? ______

02. Did you lie directly or indirectly to anyone? ______

03. What did you do to improve significant relationships with your wife, family, or friends? ______

### WHERE ARE YOU RIGHT NOW?

04. What is the lowest level you identify with on the FASTER Scale? ______

# Self-Care for Men

The topic of self-care is more often discussed as it pertains to women. To some extent, this may convey the message that men don't need self-care. This is not true.

Simply put, self-care includes all the things a person does to take care of themselves. It is the practice of doing things to preserve, improve, and protect one's health and well being. While it's important to have activities that support self-care on a regular basis, it is an essential part of navigating stressful seasons of life.

Many men were raised in an environment where self-care was linked to feminine behaviors. Even if this is not something they consciously thought, they may have developed an unconscious belief that suggests real men don't engage in or need self-care.

> "Many men want to take better care of themselves, but doing so would require becoming something society does not afford them to be—less manly."[13]

Unfortunately, this type of thinking interferes with living a long and healthy life. Consider these facts:

- Men are more at risk of disease, injury, and death compared to women.[14]
- Men are three times more likely to commit suicide than women.[15]
- Men are more likely to abuse alcohol than women.[16]
- Young men are least likely to seek help for health issues, especially those from minority communities.[17]

So considering these statistics, as men, it seems important to figure out what self-care could look like for us as an integral part of our healing journey. In many cases, the things we do for self-care will be unique to us and our situation.

---

[13] Jeff Siegel, *6 Things That Keep Men From Taking Better Care of Themselves*, Psychology Today, July 20, 2022, https://www.psychologytoday.com/us/blog/self-care-men/202207/6-things-keep-men-taking-better-care-themselves.

[14] Jeff Siegel, *6 Things That Keep Men From Taking Better Care of Themselves*.

[15] Holly Hedegaard, Sally Curtin, and Margaret Warner, "Suicide mortality in the United States, 1999–2019," NCHS Data Brief, No. 398. National Center for Health Statistics. February 2021. DOI: https://dx.doi.org/10.15620/cdc:101761.

[16] Dan Bilsker, Andrea Fogarty, and Matthew Wakefield, "Critical Issues in Men's Mental Health," *The Canadian Journal of Psychiatry*, 63(9), 590–596. April 19, 2018. DOI: https://doi.org/10.1177/0706743718766052.

[17] Louise Lynch, Maggie Long, and Anne Moorhead, "Young Men, Help-Seeking, and Mental Health Services: Exploring Barriers and Solutions," *American Journal of Men's Health*, Vol. 12(1) 138–149, 2018, DOI: 10.1177/1557988315619469.

> *Self-care equates to self-love, and it brings about a positive attitude every individual needs at every point of life. A good self-care routine enhances one's ability to accomplish tasks on time which is necessary for day-to-day tasks. It boosts your confidence, makes you mentally strong, and allows for overall good health.*[18]

When making a self-care plan, think about activities you want to do on your own, as well as activities you want to do with others. While self-care is focused on taking care of yourself, sometimes, the best way to take care of yourselves is being with others.

Here are some common self-care activities for men:

- Exercising
- Having healthy sleeping habits
- Keeping a gratitude journal
- Cooking a meal for friends/family
- Developing a hobby
- Spending time in nature/hiking
- Doing devotionals
- Getting a haircut and/or shave
- Reading a book
- Having a family movie night
- Listening to music
- Taking a class
- Hanging out with friends
- Going to a movie
- Working in the yard/gardening
- Building something
- Teaching someone else how to do something

---

[18] Keith Burton, "35 Self Care Sunday Ideas for Men," *Inside 5 am*, September 25, 2021, https://inside5am.com/self-care-sunday-ideas-men/.

## MY SELF-CARE PLAN

In the following space, identify activities you would like to incorporate into your life. Indicate whether you intend to do the activity daily, weekly, bi-weekly, or monthly. Also, determine whether the activity is something you plan to do alone or with others.

| SELF-CARE ACTIVITY | I PLAN TO DO THIS... (daily, weekly, bi-weekly, monthly) | I PLAN TO INCLUDE... (my wife, kids, friends, family) |
|---|---|---|
| | | |
| | | |
| | | |
| | | |
| | | |
| | | |
| | | |
| | | |

Developing a practical self-care plan will take time and may be a work in progress. As you discover new self-care activities, add them to your plan. Learning to care for yourself equips you to better care for others.

# FASTER Scale

Circle the behaviors on the FASTER Scale that you identify with in each section.
Identify the most powerful behavior in each section and write it next to the corresponding heading.
Answer the following three questions based on your most powerful or frequent behavior.

01. How does it affect me? How do I feel in the moment?
02. How does it affect the important people in my life?
03. Why do I do this? What is the benefit for me?

## RESTORATION ____________________

*(Accepting life on God's terms, with trust, grace, mercy, vulnerability and gratitude.)* No current secrets; working to resolve problems; identifying fears and feelings; keeping commitments to meetings, prayer, family, church, people, goals, and self; being open and honest, making eye contact; increasing in relationships with God and others; true accountability.

01. ____________________
02. ____________________
03. ____________________

## FORGETTING PRIORITIES ____________________

*(Start believing the present circumstances and moving away from trusting God. Denial; flight; a change in what's important; how you spend your time, energy, and thoughts.)* Secrets; less time/energy for God, meetings, church; avoiding support and accountability people; superficial conversations; sarcasm; isolating; changes in goals; obsessed with relationships; breaking promises and commitments; neglecting family; preoccupation with material things, TV, computers, entertainment; procrastination; lying; overconfidence; bored; hiding money; image management; seeking to control situations and other people.

01. ____________________
____________________
02. ____________________
____________________
03. ____________________
____________________

## ANXIETY

*(Consumed by negative thoughts and undefined fear; getting energy from emotions.)* Worry, using profanity, being fearful; being resentful; replaying old, negative thoughts; perfectionism; judging other's motives; making goals and lists that you can't complete; mind reading; fantasy, codependent, rescuing; sleep problems, trouble concentrating, seeking/creating drama; gossip; using over-the-counter medication for pain, sleep or weight control; flirting.

01. ____________________

02. ____________________

03. ____________________

## SPEEDING UP

*(Trying to outrun the anxiety which is usually the first sign of depression.)* Super busy and always in a hurry (finding good reason to justify the work); workaholic; can't relax; avoiding slowing down; feeling driven; can't turn off thoughts; skipping meals; binge eating (usually at night); overspending; can't identify own feelings/needs; repetitive negative thoughts; irritable; dramatic mood swings; too much caffeine; over exercising; nervousness; difficulty being alone and/or with people; difficulty listening to others; making excuses for having to "do it all."

01. ____________________

02. ____________________

03. ____________________

## TICKED OFF

*(Getting adrenaline high on anger and aggression.)* Procrastination causing crisis in money, work, and relationships; increased sarcasm; black and white (all or nothing) thinking; feeling alone; nobody understands; overreacting, road rage; constant resentments; pushing others away; increasing isolation; blaming; arguing; irrational thinking; can't take criticism; defensive; people avoiding you; needing to be right; digestive problems; headaches; obsessive (stuck) thoughts; can't forgive; feeling superior; using intimidation.

01. ______________________________________________

______________________________________________

02. ______________________________________________

______________________________________________

03. ______________________________________________

______________________________________________

## EXHAUSTED ______________________________________________

*(Loss of physical and emotional energy; coming off the adrenaline high, and the onset of depression.)* Depressed; panicked; confused; hopelessness; sleeping too much or too little; can't cope; overwhelmed; crying for "no reason"; can't think; forgetful; pessimistic; helpless; tired; numb; wanting to run; constant cravings for old coping behaviors; thinking of using sex, drugs, or alcohol; seeking old unhealthy people and places; really isolating; people angry with you; self abuse; suicidal thoughts; spontaneous crying; no goals; survival mode; not returning phone calls; missing work; irritability; no appetite.

01. ______________________________________________

______________________________________________

02. ______________________________________________

______________________________________________

03. ______________________________________________

______________________________________________

## RELAPSE ______________________________________________

*(Returning to the place you swore you would never go again. Coping with life on your terms. You sitting in the driver's seat instead of God.)* Giving up and giving in; out of control; lost in your addiction; lying to yourself and others; feeling you just can't manage without your coping behaviors, at least for now. The result is the reinforcement of shame, guilt and condemnation; and feelings of abandonment and being alone.

01. ______________________________________________

______________________________________________

02. ______________________________________________

______________________________________________

03. ______________________________________________

______________________________________________

# Commitment To Change

Complete the Commitment to Change prior to your next group meeting.

Keep in mind, your Commitment to Change is often directly connected to the lowest level reached on the FASTER Scale. Healing happens best when we are fully aware of the challenges we face and take proactive steps to create change.

## LET'S PLAN FOR NEXT WEEK

### Commitment to change: what area do you need to change or what challenge are you facing this week?

- Double bind: what will it cost you if you change? If you don't change?
- How does this potential for change make you feel?
- What is your plan to maintain restoration regarding these changes?

### Who will you share your commitment with this week?

### What are the details of your accountability? What questions should they ask you?

**BE PREPARED TO SHARE YOUR ANSWERS IN THIS CHAPTER WITH THE GUYS IN YOUR GROUP.**

# STAGE II
# WRAP UP

## What do you think?

> Be intentional about journaling. Set aside specific time to sit and wait before the Lord. Listen to the Holy Spirit. Write about what God is saying to you and/or what you see Him doing in your life through Stage II of this journey.

# Progress, Not Perfection

Where are you making progress in your goals and overall healing? Noticing these small areas of improvement empower us to keep moving forward. It's the small consistent steps toward health that lead us to lifelong healing.

| ISSUE | PERFECTION | WHERE I STARTED | PROGRESS |
|---|---|---|---|
| | | | |

What can you do this week to make progress toward your goal?

| ISSUE | PERFECTION | WHERE I STARTED | PROGRESS |
|---|---|---|---|
| | | | |

What can you do this week to make progress toward your goal?

| ISSUE | PERFECTION | WHERE I STARTED | PROGRESS |
| --- | --- | --- | --- |
| | | | |

What can you do this week to make progress toward your goal?

## Thoughts & Feelings Awareness Log

Being intentional in connecting your thoughts and feelings is helping you become a Compassionate Warrior. Keep in mind that the slightest emotional response or reaction could lead you to a new understanding about yourself and your behaviors.

| I FELT... | ...BECAUSE I THOUGHT... |
| --- | --- |
| | |
| | |
| | |

The journaling and tools in this wrap up are for you, so you can evaluate what you're learning and keep track of the progress you're making. You don't have to share any of this with the guys in your group, but can if you want to.

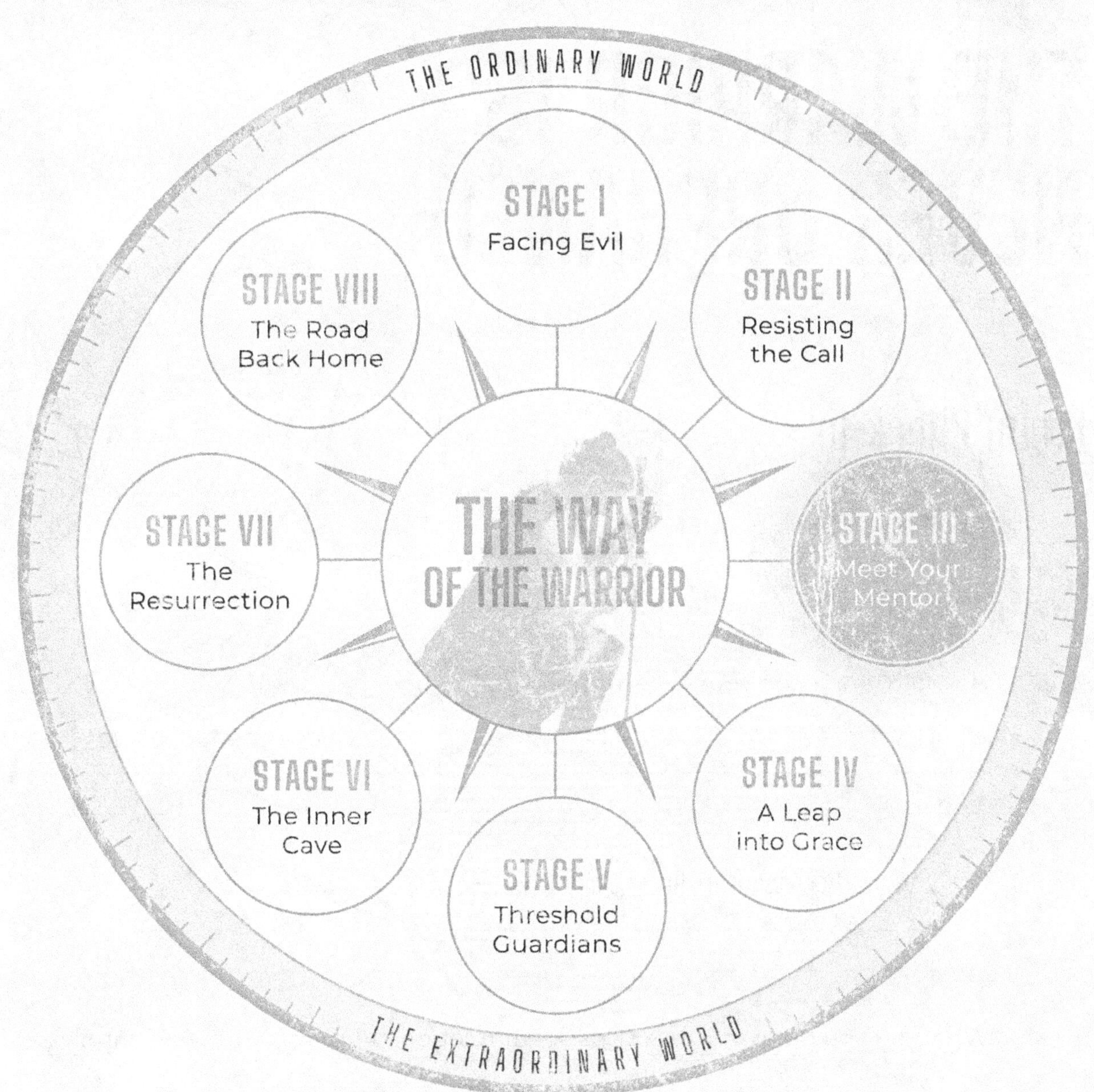


# STAGE III

## MEET YOUR MENTOR

# CHAPTER 5
# THE WARRIOR IS NEVER ORPHANED

## Group Check-In

Complete the Group Check-In 24 hours before group.

### HOW DID YOU DO LAST WEEK?

01. How did you do on your Commitment to Change? ______________________

02. Did you lie directly or indirectly to anyone? ______________________

03. What did you do to improve significant relationships with your wife, family, or friends? ______________________

### WHERE ARE YOU RIGHT NOW?

04. What is the lowest level you identify with on the FASTER Scale? ______________________

# Recognizing Triggers

As we continue to explore what lifelong health and healing looks like, it's important to be aware of our triggers: when something sparks a feeling or memory associated with a specific traumatic experience. A trigger can come from people, places, sights, sounds, smells, situations, conversations, and other forms of stimuli that creates an involuntary response. A trigger could be anything that arouses us to heightened levels of response—whether sexual in nature or emotional, such as anger, fear, and anxiety.

**Take some time to answer the following questions to better understand your triggers.**

When triggered, how do you behave? What do you do? What do you feel?

What type of situations easily trigger you?

What happened the last time you noticed being triggered this way?

Have you noticed other things that seem to happen right before you feel triggered?

Typically, what strategies do you use to get yourself back to a calm, untriggered state?

When feeling triggered, how does it affect the people around you? What do you do? What do they do?

If you could overcome one significant triggering situation and no longer feel triggered when it happens, what would it be?

# FASTER Scale

Circle the behaviors on the FASTER Scale that you identify with in each section.
Identify the most powerful behavior in each section and write it next to the corresponding heading.
Answer the following three questions based on your most powerful or frequent behavior.

01. How does it affect me? How do I feel in the moment?
02. How does it affect the important people in my life?
03. Why do I do this? What is the benefit for me?

## RESTORATION ______

*(Accepting life on God's terms, with trust, grace, mercy, vulnerability and gratitude.)* No current secrets; working to resolve problems; identifying fears and feelings; keeping commitments to meetings, prayer, family, church, people, goals, and self; being open and honest, making eye contact; increasing in relationships with God and others; true accountability.

01. ______
02. ______
03. ______

## FORGETTING PRIORITIES ______

*(Start believing the present circumstances and moving away from trusting God. Denial; flight; a change in what's important; how you spend your time, energy, and thoughts.)* Secrets; less time/energy for God, meetings, church; avoiding support and accountability people; superficial conversations; sarcasm; isolating; changes in goals; obsessed with relationships; breaking promises and commitments; neglecting family; preoccupation with material things, TV, computers, entertainment; procrastination; lying; overconfidence; bored; hiding money; image management; seeking to control situations and other people.

01. ______
______
02. ______
______
03. ______
______

## ANXIETY

*(Consumed by negative thoughts and undefined fear; getting energy from emotions.)* Worry, using profanity, being fearful; being resentful; replaying old, negative thoughts; perfectionism; judging other's motives; making goals and lists that you can't complete; mind reading; fantasy, codependent, rescuing; sleep problems, trouble concentrating, seeking/creating drama; gossip; using over-the-counter medication for pain, sleep or weight control; flirting.

01. ________________________

02. ________________________

03. ________________________

## SPEEDING UP

*(Trying to outrun the anxiety which is usually the first sign of depression.)* Super busy and always in a hurry (finding good reason to justify the work); workaholic; can't relax; avoiding slowing down; feeling driven; can't turn off thoughts; skipping meals; binge eating (usually at night); overspending; can't identify own feelings/needs; repetitive negative thoughts; irritable; dramatic mood swings; too much caffeine; over exercising; nervousness; difficulty being alone and/or with people; difficulty listening to others; making excuses for having to "do it all."

01. ________________________

02. ________________________

03. ________________________

## TICKED OFF

*(Getting adrenaline high on anger and aggression.)* Procrastination causing crisis in money, work, and relationships; increased sarcasm; black and white (all or nothing) thinking; feeling alone; nobody understands; overreacting, road rage; constant resentments; pushing others away; increasing isolation; blaming; arguing; irrational thinking; can't take criticism; defensive; people avoiding you; needing to be right; digestive problems; headaches; obsessive (stuck) thoughts; can't forgive; feeling superior; using intimidation.

01. ______________________________

______________________________

02. ______________________________

______________________________

03. ______________________________

______________________________

## EXHAUSTED ______________________________

*(Loss of physical and emotional energy; coming off the adrenaline high, and the onset of depression.)* Depressed; panicked; confused; hopelessness; sleeping too much or too little; can't cope; overwhelmed; crying for "no reason"; can't think; forgetful; pessimistic; helpless; tired; numb; wanting to run; constant cravings for old coping behaviors; thinking of using sex, drugs, or alcohol; seeking old unhealthy people and places; really isolating; people angry with you; self abuse; suicidal thoughts; spontaneous crying; no goals; survival mode; not returning phone calls; missing work; irritability; no appetite.

01. ______________________________

______________________________

02. ______________________________

______________________________

03. ______________________________

______________________________

## RELAPSE ______________________________

*(Returning to the place you swore you would never go again. Coping with life on your terms. You sitting in the driver's seat instead of God.)* Giving up and giving in; out of control; lost in your addiction; lying to yourself and others; feeling you just can't manage without your coping behaviors, at least for now. The result is the reinforcement of shame, guilt and condemnation; and feelings of abandonment and being alone.

01. ______________________________

______________________________

02. ______________________________

______________________________

03. ______________________________

______________________________

# Commitment To Change

Complete the Commitment to Change prior to your next group meeting.

Keep in mind, your Commitment to Change is often directly connected to the lowest level reached on the FASTER Scale. Healing happens best when we are fully aware of the challenges we face and take proactive steps to create change.

## LET'S PLAN FOR NEXT WEEK

### Commitment to change: what area do you need to change or what challenge are you facing this week?

- Double bind: what will it cost you if you change? If you don't change?
- How does this potential for change make you feel?
- What is your plan to maintain restoration regarding these changes?

### Who will you share your commitment with this week?

### What are the details of your accountability? What questions should they ask you?

### BE PREPARED TO SHARE YOUR ANSWERS IN THIS CHAPTER WITH THE GUYS IN YOUR GROUP.

CHAPTER 6

# THE MENTORED WARRIOR BECOMES THE MENTOR

## Group Check-In

Complete the Group Check-In 24 hours before group.

### HOW DID YOU DO LAST WEEK?

01. How did you do on your Commitment to Change? ____________________

02. Did you lie directly or indirectly to anyone? ____________________

03. What did you do to improve significant relationships with your wife, family, or friends? ____________________

### WHERE ARE YOU RIGHT NOW?

04. What is the lowest level you identify with on the FASTER Scale? ____________________

# Understanding Communication Styles

The way we communicate with others is important when it comes to relationships. We may not think of it this way, but if we're experiencing any stress or conflict in our relationships, being able to effectively communicate in order to resolve the issue is essential for the health of the relationship. When it comes to navigating relationships, it can be helpful to understand our communication style.

## COMMUNICATION STYLES QUIZ[19]

Answer "Yes" or "No" to each of the following questions based on the response that seems to best describe your behaviors.

01. Do you try to push your feelings away rather than express them to others? ☐ Yes ☐ No
02. Do you fear that expressing yourself will cause others to be angry with you or not like you? ☐ Yes ☐ No
03. Do you often say things like "I don't care" or "It doesn't matter to me" when you do care or it actually does matter? ☐ Yes ☐ No
04. Do you keep quiet or try not to rock the boat because you don't want to upset others? ☐ Yes ☐ No
05. Do you often go along with others' opinions because you don't want to be different? ☐ Yes ☐ No
06. Are you most concerned with getting your own way, regardless of how it impacts others? ☐ Yes ☐ No
07. Do you yell, swear, or use other aggressive means of communicating regularly? ☐ Yes ☐ No
08. Do your friends fear you? ☐ Yes ☐ No
09. Are you disrespectful toward others when communicating with them, not really caring if they get what they need as long as your needs are met? ☐ Yes ☐ No
10. Do you have an attitude of "my way or the highway?" Have you ever heard anyone describe you this way? ☐ Yes ☐ No
11. Do you have a tendency to be sarcastic when you feel angry? ☐ Yes ☐ No

---

19 Sheri Van Dijk, *DBT Made Simple: A Step-by-Step Guide to Dialectical Behavior Therapy* (Oakland: New Harbinger Publications, Inc., 2012), 164-168.

12. Do you tend to give people the silent treatment when you're angry with them? ☐ Yes ☐ No

13. Do you often find yourself saying one thing but thinking another, such as going along with another person's wishes even though you want to do something else? ☐ Yes ☐ No

14. Are you generally reluctant to express your emotions but find that how you feel gets expressed in other ways, like slamming doors or other aggressive behaviors? ☐ Yes ☐ No

15. Do you fear that expressing yourself will cause others to be angry with you or stop liking you, so you try to get your message across in more subtle ways? ☐ Yes ☐ No

16. Do you believe that you have a right to express your opinions and emotions? ☐ Yes ☐ No

17. When you're having a disagreement with someone, are you able to express your opinions and emotions clearly and honestly? ☐ Yes ☐ No

18. When communicating with others, do you treat them with respect while also respecting yourself? ☐ Yes ☐ No

19. Do you listen closely to what others are saying, sending them the message that you're trying to understand their perspective? ☐ Yes ☐ No

20. Do you try to negotiate with others if you have different goals, rather than being focused on getting your own needs met? ☐ Yes ☐ No

**SCORING:** Calculate the number of "Yes" responses among the following number sets. The style for which you have the most "Yes" responses is your dominant communication style.

Number of "Yes" responses:

- Questions 1 - 5: __________
- Questions 6 - 10: __________
- Questions 11 - 15: __________
- Questions 16 - 20: __________

**NOTE:** It is common for people to use different styles depending on the situation and person they're communicating with. You may also find yourself scoring similarly in two different styles. This is okay. The point of this quiz is not to diagnose how you communicate, but to increase awareness of your patterns of communication so you can choose to improve the way you communicate if needed.

## COMMUNICATION STYLES

### PASSIVE COMMUNICATION

**If you answered "Yes" to the majority of questions 1 - 5, you are a passive communicator.** Passive people often don't communicate verbally. They are more likely to bottle up their emotions instead of expressing them, fearing they will hurt others or make others uncomfortable. They don't believe their feelings or opinions matter as much as those of others. Passive communicators usually fear confrontation and believe that voicing their opinions, beliefs, or emotions will cause conflict. Their goal is usually to keep the peace, so they sit back and say little.

### AGGRESSIVE COMMUNICATION

**If you answered "Yes" to the majority of questions 6 - 10, you are an aggressive communicator.** Aggressive communicators attempt to control others. They're concerned with getting their own way, regardless of the cost. They are direct, often in a forceful, demanding, and even vicious way. They tend to leave others feeling resentful, hurt, and afraid. Although they often get what they want, it's usually at the expense of others. Sometimes, they may later feel guilty, regretful, or ashamed because of how they behaved.

### PASSIVE-AGGRESSIVE COMMUNICATION

**If you answered "Yes" to the majority of questions 11 - 15, you are a passive-aggressive communicator.** Those who have a passive-aggressive style of communication fear confrontation and don't express themselves directly, much like passive communicators. However, because of their aggressive tendencies, their goal is to get what they want but through indirect means. They often use more subtle expressions, such as sarcasm, the silent treatment, or saying they'll do something for others but then "forgetting."

### ASSERTIVE COMMUNICATION

**If you answered "Yes" to the majority of questions 15 - 20, you are an assertive communicator.** Assertive communicators express their thoughts, feelings, and beliefs in a direct and honest way that's respectful of themselves and others. While they want to get their own needs met, they also try to meet the needs of others as much as possible. They listen and negotiate, which often results in others' cooperation because they're also getting something out of it. Others often respect and value assertive communicators because this communication style makes them feel respected and valued.

People with good self-esteem tend to express themselves through assertive communication. They recognize that they have a right to express their opinions and feelings, which directly stems from their self-perception. However, people with low self-esteem can learn to be assertive in their communication style. This often improves how they feel about themselves.

What thoughts and feelings do you have after taking this Communication Quiz and discovering your dominant communication style?

What did you learn about yourself and the way you communicate?

Developing an assertive communication style can increase our self-esteem, improve relationships, and enhance interactions with others. This is helping us become a Compassionate Warrior.

# FASTER Scale

Circle the behaviors on the FASTER Scale that you identify with in each section.
Identify the most powerful behavior in each section and write it next to the corresponding heading.
Answer the following three questions based on your most powerful or frequent behavior.

01. How does it affect me? How do I feel in the moment?
02. How does it affect the important people in my life?
03. Why do I do this? What is the benefit for me?

## RESTORATION ______________________________

*(Accepting life on God's terms, with trust, grace, mercy, vulnerability and gratitude.)* No current secrets; working to resolve problems; identifying fears and feelings; keeping commitments to meetings, prayer, family, church, people, goals, and self; being open and honest, making eye contact; increasing in relationships with God and others; true accountability.

01. ______________________________
02. ______________________________
03. ______________________________

## FORGETTING PRIORITIES ______________________________

*(Start believing the present circumstances and moving away from trusting God. Denial; flight; a change in what's important; how you spend your time, energy, and thoughts.)* Secrets; less time/energy for God, meetings, church; avoiding support and accountability people; superficial conversations; sarcasm; isolating; changes in goals; obsessed with relationships; breaking promises and commitments; neglecting family; preoccupation with material things, TV, computers, entertainment; procrastination; lying; overconfidence; bored; hiding money; image management; seeking to control situations and other people.

01. ______________________________
______________________________
02. ______________________________
______________________________
03. ______________________________
______________________________

## ANXIETY

*(Consumed by negative thoughts and undefined fear; getting energy from emotions.)* Worry, using profanity, being fearful; being resentful; replaying old, negative thoughts; perfectionism; judging other's motives; making goals and lists that you can't complete; mind reading; fantasy, codependent, rescuing; sleep problems, trouble concentrating, seeking/creating drama; gossip; using over-the-counter medication for pain, sleep or weight control; flirting.

01. ______

02. ______

03. ______

## SPEEDING UP

*(Trying to outrun the anxiety which is usually the first sign of depression.)* Super busy and always in a hurry (finding good reason to justify the work); workaholic; can't relax; avoiding slowing down; feeling driven; can't turn off thoughts; skipping meals; binge eating (usually at night); overspending; can't identify own feelings/needs; repetitive negative thoughts; irritable; dramatic mood swings; too much caffeine; over exercising; nervousness; difficulty being alone and/or with people; difficulty listening to others; making excuses for having to "do it all."

01. ______

02. ______

03. ______

## TICKED OFF

*(Getting adrenaline high on anger and aggression.)* Procrastination causing crisis in money, work, and relationships; increased sarcasm; black and white (all or nothing) thinking; feeling alone; nobody understands; overreacting, road rage; constant resentments; pushing others away; increasing isolation; blaming; arguing; irrational thinking; can't take criticism; defensive; people avoiding you; needing to be right; digestive problems; headaches; obsessive (stuck) thoughts; can't forgive; feeling superior; using intimidation.

01.

02.

03.

## EXHAUSTED

*(Loss of physical and emotional energy; coming off the adrenaline high, and the onset of depression.)* Depressed; panicked; confused; hopelessness; sleeping too much or too little; can't cope; overwhelmed; crying for "no reason"; can't think; forgetful; pessimistic; helpless; tired; numb; wanting to run; constant cravings for old coping behaviors; thinking of using sex, drugs, or alcohol; seeking old unhealthy people and places; really isolating; people angry with you; self abuse; suicidal thoughts; spontaneous crying; no goals; survival mode; not returning phone calls; missing work; irritability; no appetite.

01.

02.

03.

## RELAPSE

*(Returning to the place you swore you would never go again. Coping with life on your terms. You sitting in the driver's seat instead of God.)* Giving up and giving in; out of control; lost in your addiction; lying to yourself and others; feeling you just can't manage without your coping behaviors, at least for now. The result is the reinforcement of shame, guilt and condemnation; and feelings of abandonment and being alone.

01.

02.

03.

# Commitment To Change

Complete the Commitment to Change prior to your next group meeting.

Keep in mind, your Commitment to Change is often directly connected to the lowest level reached on the FASTER Scale. Healing happens best when we are fully aware of the challenges we face and take proactive steps to create change.

## LET'S PLAN FOR NEXT WEEK

Commitment to change: what area do you need to change or what challenge are you facing this week?

- Double bind: what will it cost you if you change? If you don't change?
- How does this potential for change make you feel?
- What is your plan to maintain restoration regarding these changes?

Who will you share your commitment with this week?

What are the details of your accountability? What questions should they ask you?

BE PREPARED TO SHARE YOUR ANSWERS IN THIS CHAPTER WITH THE GUYS IN YOUR GROUP.

STAGE III

# WRAP UP

## What do you think?

Spend time journaling. As mentioned, writing by hand promotes learning and creates positive brain change. At this point in your journey, how do you see God meeting you exactly where you're at? In what ways is He giving you what you need to sustain your health and healing?

# Progress, Not Perfection

Keeping track of our progress throughout this journey often reveals something about ourselves. When we focus too much on where we want to be, and are not there yet, it can be discouraging. So focusing on our progress, even the smallest things, can make a huge difference in keeping our momentum going. In what areas are you making progress?

| ISSUE | PERFECTION | WHERE I STARTED | PROGRESS |
| --- | --- | --- | --- |
| | | | |

What can you do this week to make progress toward your goal?

| ISSUE | PERFECTION | WHERE I STARTED | PROGRESS |
| --- | --- | --- | --- |
| | | | |

What can you do this week to make progress toward your goal?

| ISSUE | PERFECTION | WHERE I STARTED | PROGRESS |
|---|---|---|---|
| | | | |

What can you do this week to make progress toward your goal?

## Thoughts & Feelings Awareness Log

Continue to work on identifying your thoughts and feelings and how they are contributing to your behaviors. The better we get at recognizing why we feel a specific way and the associated thought process, the more proactive we will become at taking our thoughts captive (2 Corinthians 10:5).

| I FELT… | …BECAUSE I THOUGHT… |
|---|---|
| | |
| | |
| | |

The journaling and tools in this wrap up are for you, so you can evaluate what you're learning and keep track of the progress you're making. You don't have to share any of this with the guys in your group, but can if you want to.

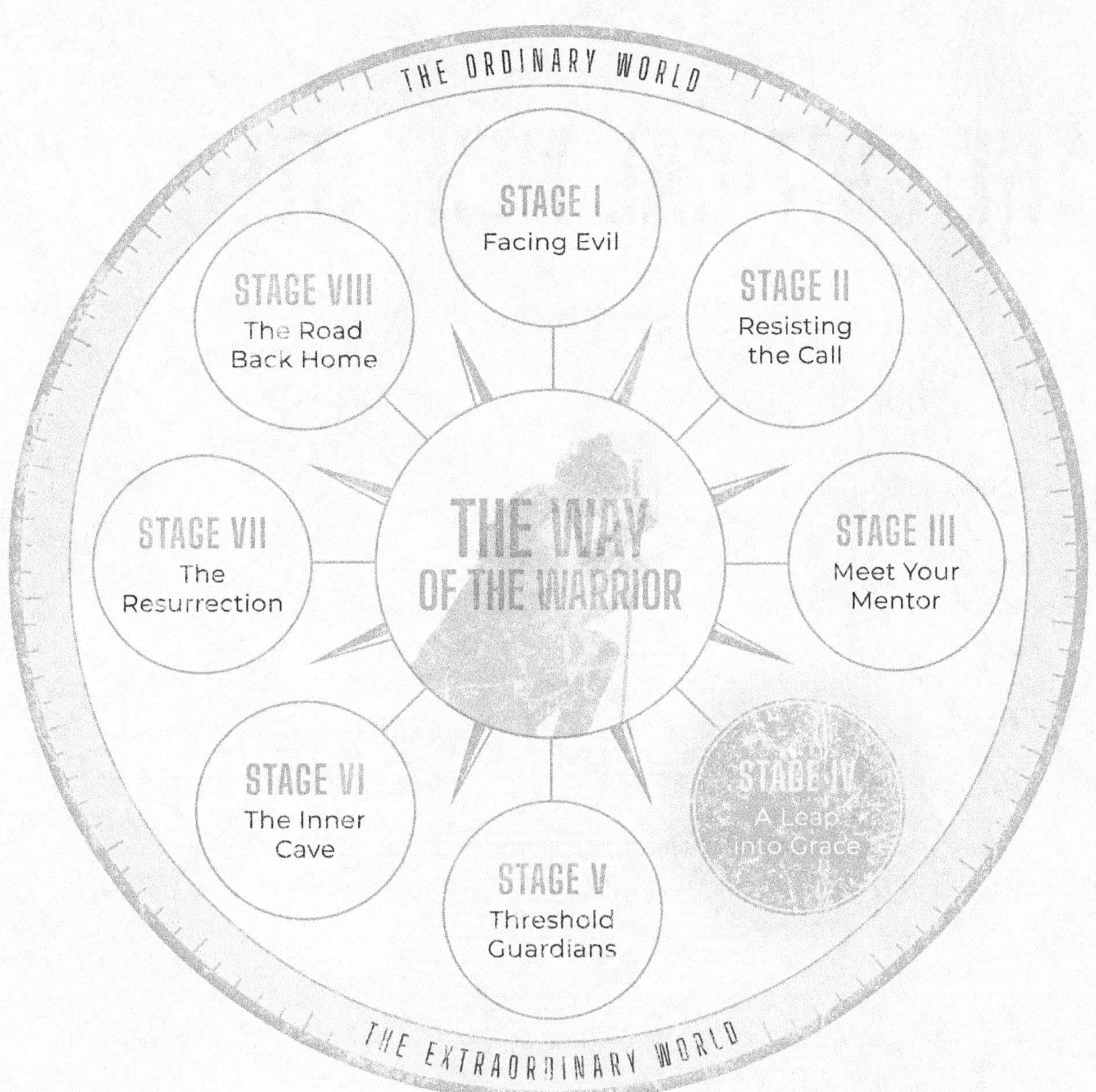


# STAGE IV

## A RADICAL LIFE-ALTERING LEAP INTO GRACE

CHAPTER 7

# THE CRITICAL NEXT STEP

## Group Check-In

Complete the Group Check-In 24 hours before group.

### HOW DID YOU DO LAST WEEK?

01. How did you do on your Commitment to Change? ______

02. Did you lie directly or indirectly to anyone? ______

03. What did you do to improve significant relationships with your wife, family, or friends? ______

### WHERE ARE YOU RIGHT NOW?

04. What is the lowest level you identify with on the FASTER Scale? ______

# A Balanced Life

Creating balance in our lives takes a unique approach. Some of us live our lives in go-mode: we are on the move 24/7 and barely stop to sleep, eat, and relax. Some of us take a slower approach to life: we take a more analytical and deliberate approach to the task, but sometimes miss opportunities. And some of us are in between: adapting to the speed of life, but never having time to enjoy the journey.

Having a balanced life happens when we can intentionally give time and space to the key areas of our lives. For now, let's focus on these four areas: physical, emotional, relational, and spiritual. If one or more of these areas is not well attended to, we become out of balance.

> Before we go any further, identify where you're at in these areas. Place a number between 0 and 10, indicating where you think you're at today. On this scale, 0 reflects "the worst I've ever been," 3 reflects "getting better," 5 reflects "good," 7 reflects "great," and 10 reflects "the best I've ever been."[20]

- Marriage/Romantic relationship ........ ______
- Mental/Emotional health ........ ______
- Career/Employment ........ ______
- Recreation/Hobbies ........ ______
- Spiritual life ........ ______
- Physical health ........ ______
- Friendships/Social life ........ ______
- Physical environment (home, car, etc.) ........ ______
- Church/Religious participation ........ ______
- Extended family ........ ______
- Relationships with children (list each separately)
  - ______________ ........ ______
  - ______________ ........ ______
  - ______________ ........ ______
  - ______________ ........ ______

Hopefully this has helped you see the areas where you're doing well and the areas that may need some improvement.

[20] Jeff Riggenbach, *The CBT Toolbox: A Workbook for Clients and Clinicians* (Eau Claire: Premier Publishing and Media, 2013), 67.

**Note:** If you scored 0 in several areas and want to further investigate this, counseling might be a good option for you. Contact Pure Desire at 503-489-0230 or visit puredesire.org/counseling/ for more information.

**Let's dig a little deeper. The choice is yours: either pick 1-3 questions in each category to answer OR, if you've identified one category that needs improvement, answer all the questions in that category.**

# Physical Health

How are your eating habits? Do you eat three meals a day or are you more of a grazer? Are you underweight or overweight? Do you drink enough water?

Are you getting enough sleep each night? Do you fall asleep easily and stay asleep? Do you take medication to help sleep at night?

Do you get enough exercise? What is your exercise routine: daily, weekly? What prevents you from getting regular exercise?

What is one healthy change you could make to improve your physical health?

# Emotional Health

What negative emotions do you experience on a regular basis?

What strategies have you used to minimize your negative emotions? What has worked? What does not work?

What activities, hobbies, and interests do you enjoy that bring about positive emotions and bring greater balance to your overall emotional health?

What is one healthy change you could make to improve your emotional health?

# Relational Health

Who in your life do you have the best relationship with? What do you enjoy most about this relationship?

Who in your life do you have the most turbulent relationship with? What factors influence the conflict you experience with this person?

List the people in your life who bring out the best in you and offer ongoing support and encouragement on a regular basis. How do they help you?

What is one healthy change you could make to improve your relational health?

## Spiritual Health

When you think about God, what thoughts, feelings, and images come to mind?

How do you incorporate faith/spirituality into your life?

How has your faith and relationship with God contributed to who you are today?

What is one healthy change you could make to improve your spiritual health?

Bringing balance to our lives will take intention and time. As we continue to invest in and attend to these various areas, we will become more balanced and experience overall health. This is what our healing journey is all about.

# FASTER Scale

Circle the behaviors on the FASTER Scale that you identify with in each section.
Identify the most powerful behavior in each section and write it next to the corresponding heading.
Answer the following three questions based on your most powerful or frequent behavior.

01. How does it affect me? How do I feel in the moment?
02. How does it affect the important people in my life?
03. Why do I do this? What is the benefit for me?

## RESTORATION ____________________

*(Accepting life on God's terms, with trust, grace, mercy, vulnerability and gratitude.)* No current secrets; working to resolve problems; identifying fears and feelings; keeping commitments to meetings, prayer, family, church, people, goals, and self; being open and honest, making eye contact; increasing in relationships with God and others; true accountability.

01. ____________________
02. ____________________
03. ____________________

## FORGETTING PRIORITIES ____________________

*(Start believing the present circumstances and moving away from trusting God. Denial; flight; a change in what's important; how you spend your time, energy, and thoughts.)* Secrets; less time/energy for God, meetings, church; avoiding support and accountability people; superficial conversations; sarcasm; isolating; changes in goals; obsessed with relationships; breaking promises and commitments; neglecting family; preoccupation with material things, TV, computers, entertainment; procrastination; lying; overconfidence; bored; hiding money; image management; seeking to control situations and other people.

01. ____________________
____________________
02. ____________________
____________________
03. ____________________
____________________

## ANXIETY

*(Consumed by negative thoughts and undefined fear; getting energy from emotions.)* Worry, using profanity, being fearful; being resentful; replaying old, negative thoughts; perfectionism; judging other's motives; making goals and lists that you can't complete; mind reading; fantasy, codependent, rescuing; sleep problems, trouble concentrating, seeking/creating drama; gossip; using over-the-counter medication for pain, sleep or weight control; flirting.

01. ______________________________

02. ______________________________

03. ______________________________

## SPEEDING UP

*(Trying to outrun the anxiety which is usually the first sign of depression.)* Super busy and always in a hurry (finding good reason to justify the work); workaholic; can't relax; avoiding slowing down; feeling driven; can't turn off thoughts; skipping meals; binge eating (usually at night); overspending; can't identify own feelings/needs; repetitive negative thoughts; irritable; dramatic mood swings; too much caffeine; over exercising; nervousness; difficulty being alone and/or with people; difficulty listening to others; making excuses for having to "do it all."

01. ______________________________

02. ______________________________

03. ______________________________

## TICKED OFF

*(Getting adrenaline high on anger and aggression.)* Procrastination causing crisis in money, work, and relationships; increased sarcasm; black and white (all or nothing) thinking; feeling alone; nobody understands; overreacting, road rage; constant resentments; pushing others away; increasing isolation; blaming; arguing; irrational thinking; can't take criticism; defensive; people avoiding you; needing to be right; digestive problems; headaches; obsessive (stuck) thoughts; can't forgive; feeling superior; using intimidation.

01. ______________________________________________

______________________________________________

02. ______________________________________________

______________________________________________

03. ______________________________________________

______________________________________________

## EXHAUSTED

*(Loss of physical and emotional energy; coming off the adrenaline high, and the onset of depression.)* Depressed; panicked; confused; hopelessness; sleeping too much or too little; can't cope; overwhelmed; crying for "no reason"; can't think; forgetful; pessimistic; helpless; tired; numb; wanting to run; constant cravings for old coping behaviors; thinking of using sex, drugs, or alcohol; seeking old unhealthy people and places; really isolating; people angry with you; self abuse; suicidal thoughts; spontaneous crying; no goals; survival mode; not returning phone calls; missing work; irritability; no appetite.

01. ______________________________________________

______________________________________________

02. ______________________________________________

______________________________________________

03. ______________________________________________

______________________________________________

## RELAPSE

*(Returning to the place you swore you would never go again. Coping with life on your terms. You sitting in the driver's seat instead of God.)* Giving up and giving in; out of control; lost in your addiction; lying to yourself and others; feeling you just can't manage without your coping behaviors, at least for now. The result is the reinforcement of shame, guilt and condemnation; and feelings of abandonment and being alone.

01. ______________________________________________

______________________________________________

02. ______________________________________________

______________________________________________

03. ______________________________________________

______________________________________________

# Commitment To Change

Complete the Commitment to Change prior to your next group meeting.

Keep in mind, your Commitment to Change is often directly connected to the lowest level reached on the FASTER Scale. Healing happens best when we are fully aware of the challenges we face and take proactive steps to create change.

## LET'S PLAN FOR NEXT WEEK

### Commitment to change: what area do you need to change or what challenge are you facing this week?

- Double bind: what will it cost you if you change? If you don't change?
- How does this potential for change make you feel?
- What is your plan to maintain restoration regarding these changes?

### Who will you share your commitment with this week?

### What are the details of your accountability? What questions should they ask you?

### BE PREPARED TO SHARE YOUR ANSWERS IN THIS CHAPTER WITH THE GUYS IN YOUR GROUP.

CHAPTER 8

# TRICKY JAKE—PART 1

## Group Check-In

Complete the Group Check-In 24 hours before group.

### HOW DID YOU DO LAST WEEK?

01. How did you do on your Commitment to Change? ______

02. Did you lie directly or indirectly to anyone? ______

03. What did you do to improve significant relationships with your wife, family, or friends? ______

### WHERE ARE YOU RIGHT NOW?

04. What is the lowest level you identify with on the FASTER Scale? ______

# The Me Others See

In the chapter this week, we learned about Jacob's life and the way he schemed and deceived to get what he wanted. In many ways he pretended to be someone he was not. Within the context of the lesson this profound statement was made: **God can't bless who you pretend to be!**

Who do we pretend to be? We may not be intentionally or consciously pretending to be someone else. So let's think of it this way: who is it that we allow others to see?

This is a great question and definitely worth exploring!

**Use the following questions to gain insight into who you allow others to see.**

### What aspects of yourself do you like/want others to see?

**Personal qualities/characteristics:**

*Example: I want people to know I'm funny, energetic, and spontaneous.*

**Experiences and accomplishments:**

*Example: I like when people know that I'm a runner and have participated in several marathons.*

**Hopes and fears:**

*Example: I like people to know I'm a writer and hope to publish a novel some day. My close friends know I fear rejection and abandonment; my dad left when I was young.*

**Likes and dislikes:**

*Example: I want people to know that I like movies; all types of movies. I'm pretty transparent about the movies I don't like.*

What adjectives or phrases would you like others to use when describing you?

*Examples: honest; caring; godly; smart; a hard worker; always willing to help.*

What aspects of yourself do you not want others to know/see? Why do you want to hide these things from others?

*Example: I don't want others to know about the abuse I've experienced. I hide this from others because I feel ashamed and guilty about it.*

How do you hide or mask these things about yourself from others?

*Example: When I feel uncomfortable talking about my past, I use sarcasm or make jokes as a distraction.*

What qualities do you like to see in others that make you feel safe and allow you to show them your true, authentic self?

*Example: When others share deep parts of their past with me, it builds trust and makes me feel safe to share the hidden parts of my past with them.*

What did you learn or what observations do you have after completing this exercise?

Part of this journey requires us to look honestly at ourselves and how we show up in relationships. Becoming a Compassionate Warrior includes having compassion for ourselves and our experiences, so we can find healing and continue to reveal our true, authentic self.

# FASTER Scale

Circle the behaviors on the FASTER Scale that you identify with in each section.
Identify the most powerful behavior in each section and write it next to the corresponding heading.
Answer the following three questions based on your most powerful or frequent behavior.

01. How does it affect me? How do I feel in the moment?
02. How does it affect the important people in my life?
03. Why do I do this? What is the benefit for me?

## RESTORATION ____________________

*(Accepting life on God's terms, with trust, grace, mercy, vulnerability and gratitude.)* No current secrets; working to resolve problems; identifying fears and feelings; keeping commitments to meetings, prayer, family, church, people, goals, and self; being open and honest, making eye contact; increasing in relationships with God and others; true accountability.

01. ____________________
02. ____________________
03. ____________________

## FORGETTING PRIORITIES ____________________

*(Start believing the present circumstances and moving away from trusting God. Denial; flight; a change in what's important; how you spend your time, energy, and thoughts.)* Secrets; less time/energy for God, meetings, church; avoiding support and accountability people; superficial conversations; sarcasm; isolating; changes in goals; obsessed with relationships; breaking promises and commitments; neglecting family; preoccupation with material things, TV, computers, entertainment; procrastination; lying; overconfidence; bored; hiding money; image management; seeking to control situations and other people.

01. ____________________
____________________
02. ____________________
____________________
03. ____________________
____________________

## ANXIETY

*(Consumed by negative thoughts and undefined fear; getting energy from emotions.)* Worry, using profanity, being fearful; being resentful; replaying old, negative thoughts; perfectionism; judging other's motives; making goals and lists that you can't complete; mind reading; fantasy, codependent, rescuing; sleep problems, trouble concentrating, seeking/creating drama; gossip; using over-the-counter medication for pain, sleep or weight control; flirting.

01. __________

02. __________

03. __________

## SPEEDING UP

*(Trying to outrun the anxiety which is usually the first sign of depression.)* Super busy and always in a hurry (finding good reason to justify the work); workaholic; can't relax; avoiding slowing down; feeling driven; can't turn off thoughts; skipping meals; binge eating (usually at night); overspending; can't identify own feelings/needs; repetitive negative thoughts; irritable; dramatic mood swings; too much caffeine; over exercising; nervousness; difficulty being alone and/or with people; difficulty listening to others; making excuses for having to "do it all."

01. __________

02. __________

03. __________

## TICKED OFF

*(Getting adrenaline high on anger and aggression.)* Procrastination causing crisis in money, work, and relationships; increased sarcasm; black and white (all or nothing) thinking; feeling alone; nobody understands; overreacting, road rage; constant resentments; pushing others away; increasing isolation; blaming; arguing; irrational thinking; can't take criticism; defensive; people avoiding you; needing to be right; digestive problems; headaches; obsessive (stuck) thoughts; can't forgive; feeling superior; using intimidation.

01. ______________________________________________

______________________________________________

02. ______________________________________________

______________________________________________

03. ______________________________________________

______________________________________________

## EXHAUSTED ______________________________________________

*(Loss of physical and emotional energy; coming off the adrenaline high, and the onset of depression.)* Depressed; panicked; confused; hopelessness; sleeping too much or too little; can't cope; overwhelmed; crying for "no reason"; can't think; forgetful; pessimistic; helpless; tired; numb; wanting to run; constant cravings for old coping behaviors; thinking of using sex, drugs, or alcohol; seeking old unhealthy people and places; really isolating; people angry with you; self abuse; suicidal thoughts; spontaneous crying; no goals; survival mode; not returning phone calls; missing work; irritability; no appetite.

01. ______________________________________________

______________________________________________

02. ______________________________________________

______________________________________________

03. ______________________________________________

______________________________________________

## RELAPSE ______________________________________________

*(Returning to the place you swore you would never go again. Coping with life on your terms. You sitting in the driver's seat instead of God.)* Giving up and giving in; out of control; lost in your addiction; lying to yourself and others; feeling you just can't manage without your coping behaviors, at least for now. The result is the reinforcement of shame, guilt and condemnation; and feelings of abandonment and being alone.

01. ______________________________________________

______________________________________________

02. ______________________________________________

______________________________________________

03. ______________________________________________

______________________________________________

# Commitment To Change

Complete the Commitment to Change prior to your next group meeting.

Keep in mind, your Commitment to Change is often directly connected to the lowest level reached on the FASTER Scale. Healing happens best when we are fully aware of the challenges we face and take proactive steps to create change.

## LET'S PLAN FOR NEXT WEEK

Commitment to change: what area do you need to change or what challenge are you facing this week?

- Double bind: what will it cost you if you change? If you don't change?
- How does this potential for change make you feel?
- What is your plan to maintain restoration regarding these changes?

Who will you share your commitment with this week?

What are the details of your accountability? What questions should they ask you?

BE PREPARED TO SHARE YOUR ANSWERS IN THIS CHAPTER WITH THE GUYS IN YOUR GROUP.

# CHAPTER 9
# TRICKY JAKE—PART 2

## Group Check-In

Complete the Group Check-In 24 hours before group.

### HOW DID YOU DO LAST WEEK?

01. How did you do on your Commitment to Change? ______

02. Did you lie directly or indirectly to anyone? ______

03. What did you do to improve significant relationships with your wife, family, or friends? ______

### WHERE ARE YOU RIGHT NOW?

04. What is the lowest level you identify with on the FASTER Scale? ______

# Identifying Feelings

Many men struggle with identifying their feelings. This happens for several reasons: they weren't raised in an environment where feelings were talked about and expressed; through experience, they've learned feelings are not safe and not useful; talking about feelings makes others uncomfortable so it's best to keep feelings to ourselves; they've been told, men don't talk about their feelings; and a million other reasons that indicate men and feelings should never mix.

The glaring problem with this is that men do have feelings. Men are emotional. Yet we are rarely taught about emotions, let alone taught how to express our feelings in a healthy way.

Being able to recognize what we're feeling when we're feeling it raises our emotional awareness. Sometimes we may not be able to name what we're feeling, but we notice a shift in how we physically feel. We may experience an upset stomach because we feel anxious. Or our heart might start racing because we feel irritated or angry. Or we might get a headache because we feel stressed. Pay attention to these physical symptoms as well.

Keep in mind, feelings are not good or bad, right or wrong. They are information for us; an indication that we need to pay attention to something.

On the following chart, keep track of your feelings this week.[21] Throughout each day, pay attention to the feelings you experience (emotionally and physically) and place a check mark in the corresponding feelings row.

Start and end your "week" as it aligns with your group meeting. For example, if your group meets on Thursday nights, then your "week" will start on Friday and go through Thursday.

[21] Jeff Riggenbach, *The CBT Toolbox: A Workbook for Clients and Clinicians* (Eau Claire: Premier Publishing and Media, 2013), 15.

# Feelings Chart

| TYPE OF FEELING | MON | TUES | WED | THURS | FRI | SAT | SUN |
|---|---|---|---|---|---|---|---|
| Happy | | | | | | | |
| Sad | | | | | | | |
| Excited | | | | | | | |
| Angry | | | | | | | |
| Stressed | | | | | | | |
| Proud | | | | | | | |
| Encouraged | | | | | | | |
| Regretful | | | | | | | |
| Confident | | | | | | | |
| Guilty | | | | | | | |
| Playful | | | | | | | |
| Anxious | | | | | | | |
| Grateful | | | | | | | |
| Gloomy | | | | | | | |
| Loved | | | | | | | |
| Hopeful | | | | | | | |
| Jealous | | | | | | | |
| Curious | | | | | | | |
| Irritated | | | | | | | |
| Peaceful | | | | | | | |
| Ashamed | | | | | | | |
| Energetic | | | | | | | |

**After tracking your feelings throughout the week, answer the following questions:**

What feeling(s) showed up with the greatest frequency?

What information does this give you? What might you need to pay attention to in your life right now?

Was this a typical week for you or were there extra things going on in your life?

Raising awareness of our emotional health is an important part of our next level healing. The more comfortable we get with identifying our feelings, the more equipped we are at recognizing them in others. This is the goal of emotional growth.

# FASTER Scale

Circle the behaviors on the FASTER Scale that you identify with in each section.
Identify the most powerful behavior in each section and write it next to the corresponding heading.
Answer the following three questions based on your most powerful or frequent behavior.

01. How does it affect me? How do I feel in the moment?
02. How does it affect the important people in my life?
03. Why do I do this? What is the benefit for me?

## RESTORATION ______________________

*(Accepting life on God's terms, with trust, grace, mercy, vulnerability and gratitude.)* No current secrets; working to resolve problems; identifying fears and feelings; keeping commitments to meetings, prayer, family, church, people, goals, and self; being open and honest, making eye contact; increasing in relationships with God and others; true accountability.

01. ______________________
02. ______________________
03. ______________________

## FORGETTING PRIORITIES ______________________

*(Start believing the present circumstances and moving away from trusting God. Denial; flight; a change in what's important; how you spend your time, energy, and thoughts.)* Secrets; less time/energy for God, meetings, church; avoiding support and accountability people; superficial conversations; sarcasm; isolating; changes in goals; obsessed with relationships; breaking promises and commitments; neglecting family; preoccupation with material things, TV, computers, entertainment; procrastination; lying; overconfidence; bored; hiding money; image management; seeking to control situations and other people.

01. ______________________
______________________
02. ______________________
______________________
03. ______________________
______________________

## ANXIETY

*(Consumed by negative thoughts and undefined fear; getting energy from emotions.)* Worry, using profanity, being fearful; being resentful; replaying old, negative thoughts; perfectionism; judging other's motives; making goals and lists that you can't complete; mind reading; fantasy, codependent, rescuing; sleep problems, trouble concentrating, seeking/creating drama; gossip; using over-the-counter medication for pain, sleep or weight control; flirting.

01. ______________________________

02. ______________________________

03. ______________________________

## SPEEDING UP

*(Trying to outrun the anxiety which is usually the first sign of depression.)* Super busy and always in a hurry (finding good reason to justify the work); workaholic; can't relax; avoiding slowing down; feeling driven; can't turn off thoughts; skipping meals; binge eating (usually at night); overspending; can't identify own feelings/needs; repetitive negative thoughts; irritable; dramatic mood swings; too much caffeine; over exercising; nervousness; difficulty being alone and/or with people; difficulty listening to others; making excuses for having to "do it all."

01. ______________________________

02. ______________________________

03. ______________________________

## TICKED OFF

*(Getting adrenaline high on anger and aggression.)* Procrastination causing crisis in money, work, and relationships; increased sarcasm; black and white (all or nothing) thinking; feeling alone; nobody understands; overreacting, road rage; constant resentments; pushing others away; increasing isolation; blaming; arguing; irrational thinking; can't take criticism; defensive; people avoiding you; needing to be right; digestive problems; headaches; obsessive (stuck) thoughts; can't forgive; feeling superior; using intimidation.

01. ______________________________________________

______________________________________________

02. ______________________________________________

______________________________________________

03. ______________________________________________

______________________________________________

## EXHAUSTED

*(Loss of physical and emotional energy; coming off the adrenaline high, and the onset of depression.)* Depressed; panicked; confused; hopelessness; sleeping too much or too little; can't cope; overwhelmed; crying for "no reason"; can't think; forgetful; pessimistic; helpless; tired; numb; wanting to run; constant cravings for old coping behaviors; thinking of using sex, drugs, or alcohol; seeking old unhealthy people and places; really isolating; people angry with you; self abuse; suicidal thoughts; spontaneous crying; no goals; survival mode; not returning phone calls; missing work; irritability; no appetite.

01. ______________________________________________

______________________________________________

02. ______________________________________________

______________________________________________

03. ______________________________________________

______________________________________________

## RELAPSE

*(Returning to the place you swore you would never go again. Coping with life on your terms. You sitting in the driver's seat instead of God.)* Giving up and giving in; out of control; lost in your addiction; lying to yourself and others; feeling you just can't manage without your coping behaviors, at least for now. The result is the reinforcement of shame, guilt and condemnation; and feelings of abandonment and being alone.

01. ______________________________________________

______________________________________________

02. ______________________________________________

______________________________________________

03. ______________________________________________

______________________________________________

# Commitment To Change

Complete the Commitment to Change prior to your next group meeting.

Keep in mind, your Commitment to Change is often directly connected to the lowest level reached on the FASTER Scale. Healing happens best when we are fully aware of the challenges we face and take proactive steps to create change.

## LET'S PLAN FOR NEXT WEEK

### Commitment to change: what area do you need to change or what challenge are you facing this week?

- Double bind: what will it cost you if you change? If you don't change?
- How does this potential for change make you feel?
- What is your plan to maintain restoration regarding these changes?

### Who will you share your commitment with this week?

### What are the details of your accountability? What questions should they ask you?

BE PREPARED TO SHARE YOUR ANSWERS IN THIS CHAPTER WITH THE GUYS IN YOUR GROUP.

STAGE IV
# WRAP UP

## What do you think?

> As we continue to unpack what it means to be a Compassionate Warrior, it is changing us: how we see God, ourselves, and others. Journaling is a great place to explore your thoughts and feelings around these changes, what you've learned through Stage IV, and how it's impacting you and those around you.

# Progress, not Perfection

The idea that this life and this journey is about progress, not perfection is so freeing! It allows us to take our focus off ourselves and our performance and focus on the relationships we have with others. Pay attention to where you're making progress in repairing or rebuilding relationships. Even the smallest step can make a huge difference over time.

| ISSUE | PERFECTION | WHERE I STARTED | PROGRESS |
|---|---|---|---|
| | | | |

What can you do this week to make progress toward your goal?

| ISSUE | PERFECTION | WHERE I STARTED | PROGRESS |
|---|---|---|---|
| | | | |

What can you do this week to make progress toward your goal?

| ISSUE | PERFECTION | WHERE I STARTED | PROGRESS |
|---|---|---|---|
| | | | |

What can you do this week to make progress toward your goal?

## Thoughts & Feelings Awareness Log

As we become more in tune with our thoughts and feelings, and the connection between them, it changes us. We become more intentional in our relationships, better equipped to communicate our feelings in a healthy way, and more aware of the feelings of others.

| I FELT... | ...BECAUSE I THOUGHT... |
|---|---|
| | |
| | |
| | |

The journaling and tools in this wrap up are for you, so you can evaluate what you're learning and keep track of the progress you're making. You don't have to share any of this with the guys in your group, but can if you want to.

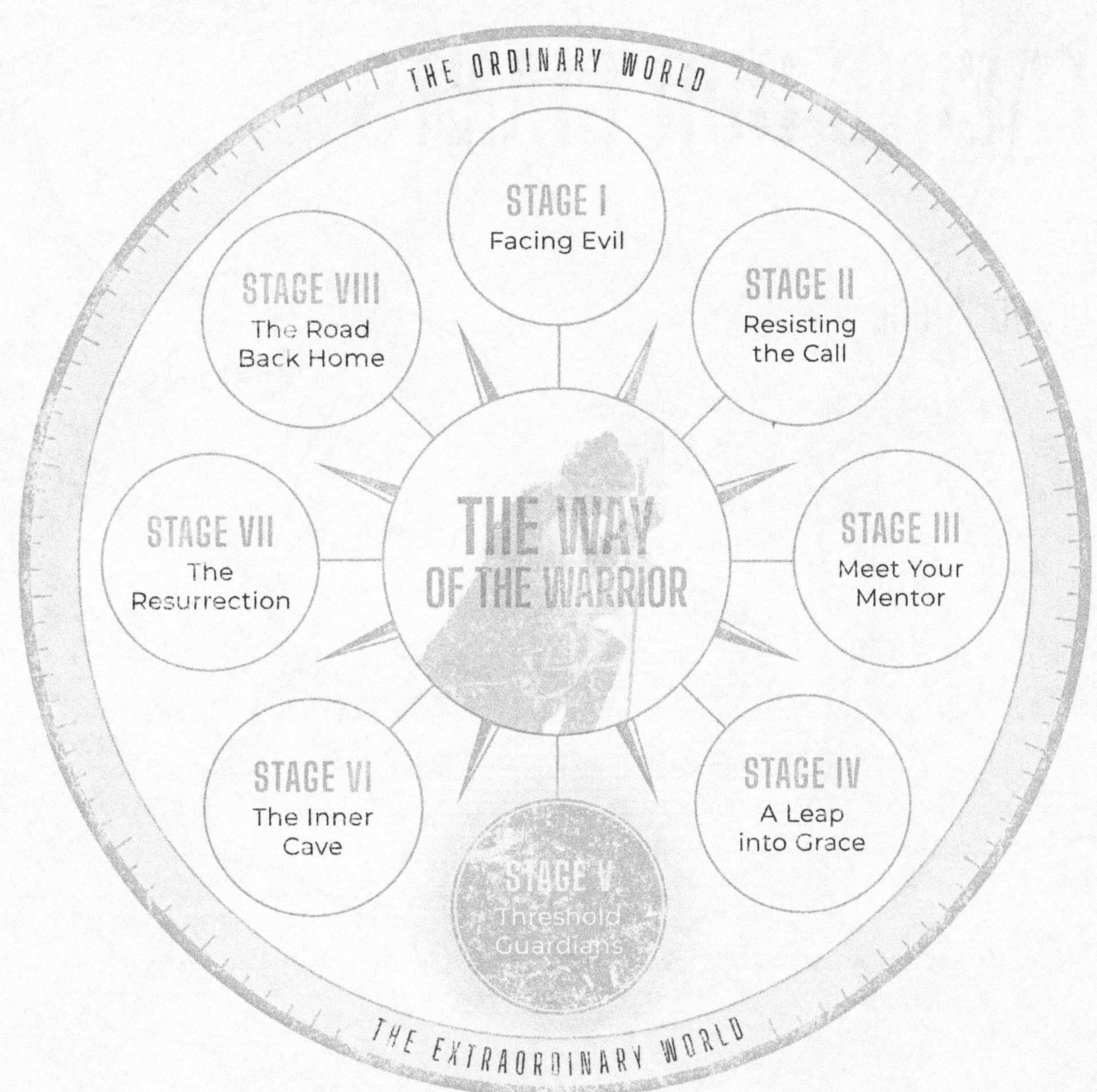


# STAGE V

## THRESHOLD GUARDIANS

CHAPTER 10

# FACING OUR GIANTS

## Group Check-In

Complete the Group Check-In 24 hours before group.

### HOW DID YOU DO LAST WEEK?

01. How did you do on your Commitment to Change? ______________________

02. Did you lie directly or indirectly to anyone? ______________________

03. What did you do to improve significant relationships with your wife, family, or friends? ______________________

### WHERE ARE YOU RIGHT NOW?

04. What is the lowest level you identify with on the FASTER Scale? ______________________

# Relationship Boundaries

One thing we learned early in our recovery journey was the need for boundaries. To some extent, we set strong boundaries around the things that could potentially lead us back to relapse. This is a very common and very broad relapse prevention strategy: don't do the things you did when you were caught up in your addiction; don't go to the places you went to when you were struggling; don't hangout with the people who played a role in your addictive behaviors. These are all sobriety 101 strategies.

Now that you've gained or are working to maintain sobriety, setting boundaries is still an important part of this healing journey, especially as it pertains to your relationship boundaries. Keep in mind: **boundaries are for you.** They reflect the decisions you've made around activities, places, and people that form a protective perimeter around how you live.

Some boundaries are fluid and only needed during the initial stages of recovery or for a period of time following relapse. Whereas other boundaries will always be there; a constant protective barrier to keep you from hurting yourself and/or others.

The further you get in your healing, you may begin to recognize a shift in the way you approach setting boundaries. At first, your boundaries may have been broad and served as guardrails around your behaviors. Now, as you continue to learn more about what it means to become a Compassionate Warrior, understanding your boundary style in relationships will help you continue to make wise decisions around your health and healing.[22]

## RELATIONSHIP BOUNDARY STYLES

People who have **porous relationship boundaries** let anyone get close to them. They are very trusting of others, even when they meet someone for the first time. They share everything about their lives and often become overly involved in the lives of others. It's very difficult for them to say "no" when others ask them to do something. They are quick to take on the opinions of others and give in to others' demands in an effort to avoid conflict. They have trouble upholding and communicating their personal values.

People who have **healthy relationship boundaries** are selective about who has access to their life. They take time to build trust in relationships and only share information about themselves as needed. They can say "no" to others without it

---

[22] Boundary Styles, TherapistAid.com, 2022, https://www.therapistaid.com/therapy-worksheet/boundary-styles.

creating stress or guilt. They provide appropriate support to others without becoming overly involved. They value their own opinions, as well as the opinions of others. They don't fear conflict and see it as a normal part of relationships. They adhere to their personal values and have no problem communicating this in relationships.

People who have **rigid relationship boundaries** keep others at a distance because they don't trust anyone. They are very guarded with their personal information. They say "no" to others most of the time. They remain detached from others; often ignoring others' opinions and pushing them away to avoid conflict. They have unwavering values and tend to be aggressive in the way they communicate with others.

Based on these brief descriptions, what is your relationship boundary style? Explain why you chose this style for yourself.

In what area(s) of your life do you have porous boundaries that are creating unhealth in relationships?

What is one thing you could do to strengthen your relationship boundaries in this area?

In what area(s) of your life do you have rigid boundaries that are creating unhealth in relationships?

If having a rigid boundary in this area is creating unhealth in relationships, what is one thing you could do to create a more healthy boundary? (Sometimes, we may have a rigid boundary in place because it keeps us from relapsing. Consider this when answering this question.)

Understanding our relationship boundary style is vital to our healing and our pursuit to becoming a Compassionate Warrior. Relationship boundaries are good and give us healthy control in our lives. They keep us safe and on the path that leads to lifelong, sustainable health.

# FASTER Scale

Circle the behaviors on the FASTER Scale that you identify with in each section.
Identify the most powerful behavior in each section and write it next to the corresponding heading.
Answer the following three questions based on your most powerful or frequent behavior.

01. How does it affect me? How do I feel in the moment?
02. How does it affect the important people in my life?
03. Why do I do this? What is the benefit for me?

## RESTORATION ______________________

*(Accepting life on God's terms, with trust, grace, mercy, vulnerability and gratitude.)* No current secrets; working to resolve problems; identifying fears and feelings; keeping commitments to meetings, prayer, family, church, people, goals, and self; being open and honest, making eye contact; increasing in relationships with God and others; true accountability.

01. ______________________
02. ______________________
03. ______________________

## FORGETTING PRIORITIES ______________________

*(Start believing the present circumstances and moving away from trusting God. Denial; flight; a change in what's important; how you spend your time, energy, and thoughts.)* Secrets; less time/energy for God, meetings, church; avoiding support and accountability people; superficial conversations; sarcasm; isolating; changes in goals; obsessed with relationships; breaking promises and commitments; neglecting family; preoccupation with material things, TV, computers, entertainment; procrastination; lying; overconfidence; bored; hiding money; image management; seeking to control situations and other people.

01. ______________________
______________________
02. ______________________
______________________
03. ______________________
______________________

## ANXIETY

*(Consumed by negative thoughts and undefined fear; getting energy from emotions.)* Worry, using profanity, being fearful; being resentful; replaying old, negative thoughts; perfectionism; judging other's motives; making goals and lists that you can't complete; mind reading; fantasy, codependent, rescuing; sleep problems, trouble concentrating, seeking/creating drama; gossip; using over-the-counter medication for pain, sleep or weight control; flirting.

01. ______________________________

02. ______________________________

03. ______________________________

## SPEEDING UP

*(Trying to outrun the anxiety which is usually the first sign of depression.)* Super busy and always in a hurry (finding good reason to justify the work); workaholic; can't relax; avoiding slowing down; feeling driven; can't turn off thoughts; skipping meals; binge eating (usually at night); overspending; can't identify own feelings/needs; repetitive negative thoughts; irritable; dramatic mood swings; too much caffeine; over exercising; nervousness; difficulty being alone and/or with people; difficulty listening to others; making excuses for having to "do it all."

01. ______________________________

02. ______________________________

03. ______________________________

## TICKED OFF

*(Getting adrenaline high on anger and aggression.)* Procrastination causing crisis in money, work, and relationships; increased sarcasm; black and white (all or nothing) thinking; feeling alone; nobody understands; overreacting, road rage; constant resentments; pushing others away; increasing isolation; blaming; arguing; irrational thinking; can't take criticism; defensive; people avoiding you; needing to be right; digestive problems; headaches; obsessive (stuck) thoughts; can't forgive; feeling superior; using intimidation.

01. ______________________________

______________________________

02. ______________________________

______________________________

03. ______________________________

______________________________

## EXHAUSTED

*(Loss of physical and emotional energy; coming off the adrenaline high, and the onset of depression.)* Depressed; panicked; confused; hopelessness; sleeping too much or too little; can't cope; overwhelmed; crying for "no reason"; can't think; forgetful; pessimistic; helpless; tired; numb; wanting to run; constant cravings for old coping behaviors; thinking of using sex, drugs, or alcohol; seeking old unhealthy people and places; really isolating; people angry with you; self abuse; suicidal thoughts; spontaneous crying; no goals; survival mode; not returning phone calls; missing work; irritability; no appetite.

01. ______________________________

______________________________

02. ______________________________

______________________________

03. ______________________________

______________________________

## RELAPSE

*(Returning to the place you swore you would never go again. Coping with life on your terms. You sitting in the driver's seat instead of God.)* Giving up and giving in; out of control; lost in your addiction; lying to yourself and others; feeling you just can't manage without your coping behaviors, at least for now. The result is the reinforcement of shame, guilt and condemnation; and feelings of abandonment and being alone.

01. ______________________________

______________________________

02. ______________________________

______________________________

03. ______________________________

______________________________

# Commitment To Change

Complete the Commitment to Change prior to your next group meeting.

Keep in mind, your Commitment to Change is often directly connected to the lowest level reached on the FASTER Scale. Healing happens best when we are fully aware of the challenges we face and take proactive steps to create change.

## LET'S PLAN FOR NEXT WEEK

### Commitment to change: what area do you need to change or what challenge are you facing this week?

- Double bind: what will it cost you if you change? If you don't change?
- How does this potential for change make you feel?
- What is your plan to maintain restoration regarding these changes?

### Who will you share your commitment with this week?

### What are the details of your accountability? What questions should they ask you?

### BE PREPARED TO SHARE YOUR ANSWERS IN THIS CHAPTER WITH THE GUYS IN YOUR GROUP.

CHAPTER 11

# THE SUPERHERO ODYSSEY—PART 1

## Group Check-In

Complete the Group Check-In 24 hours before group.

### HOW DID YOU DO LAST WEEK?

01. How did you do on your Commitment to Change? ______________________

02. Did you lie directly or indirectly to anyone? ______________________

03. What did you do to improve significant relationships with your wife, family, or friends? ______________________

### WHERE ARE YOU RIGHT NOW?

04. What is the lowest level you identify with on the FASTER Scale? ______________________

# My Identity in Christ

Scripture tells us that we were made in the image of God.[23] So it would stand to reason, since we are created in the image of God, we would have characteristics in us that reflect our heavenly Father. The same way many of us have characteristics that reflect our earthly father.

When Jesus walked the earth He was both a man and God. In His humanness, He reflected the characteristics of His heavenly Father. As a follower of Jesus, and through the Holy Spirit who dwells in us, we have the capacity to live out these characteristics in everything we do. In fact, it's our identity in Christ that gives us strength and allows us to face our "Threshold Guardians" in life.

Look up the following Scriptures and identify the various characteristics of God found in each one.

- Psalm 145:8-9 ______________________________
  ______________________________
- Psalm 145:13 ______________________________
  ______________________________
- Psalm 145:17 ______________________________
  ______________________________
- Psalm 147:5-6 ______________________________
  ______________________________
- Matthew 5:48 ______________________________
  ______________________________
- Romans 9:15 ______________________________
  ______________________________
- Romans 11:33 ______________________________
- 1 Corinthians 1:9 ______________________________
- 1 John 4:7-8 ______________________________

While we cannot be perfect this side of heaven, we can work every day to become more Christlike in our thoughts, attitudes, and actions.

---

[23] Genesis 1:26-27

From the characteristics listed, identify three that you want to improve in yourself. Next to each, explain why you chose this characteristic and how it will help you become the man God created you to be.

**Characteristic 1:** ______________________________

**Explain:** ______________________________

______________________________

______________________________

______________________________

______________________________

**Characteristic 2:** ______________________________

**Explain:** ______________________________

______________________________

______________________________

______________________________

**Characteristic 3:** ______________________________

**Explain:** ______________________________

______________________________

______________________________

______________________________

Our ability to love God, ourselves, and others comes from knowing God.

> *Dear friends, let us continue to love one another, for love comes from God. Anyone who loves is a child of God and knows God. But anyone who does not love does not know God, for God is love. God showed how much he loved us by sending his one and only Son into the world so that we might have eternal life through him. This is real love—not that we loved God, but that he loved us and sent his Son as a sacrifice to take away our sins. Dear friends, since God loved us that much, we surely ought to love each other.*
>
> 1 JOHN 4:7-11 (NLT)

We are His chosen son and an heir to share in His glory.[24] When we live with this understanding, we reflect the characteristics of God to those around us.

24 Romans 8:17.

# FASTER Scale

Circle the behaviors on the FASTER Scale that you identify with in each section.
Identify the most powerful behavior in each section and write it next to the corresponding heading.
Answer the following three questions based on your most powerful or frequent behavior.

01. How does it affect me? How do I feel in the moment?
02. How does it affect the important people in my life?
03. Why do I do this? What is the benefit for me?

## RESTORATION ______________________

*(Accepting life on God's terms, with trust, grace, mercy, vulnerability and gratitude.)* No current secrets; working to resolve problems; identifying fears and feelings; keeping commitments to meetings, prayer, family, church, people, goals, and self; being open and honest, making eye contact; increasing in relationships with God and others; true accountability.

01. ______________________
02. ______________________
03. ______________________

## FORGETTING PRIORITIES ______________________

*(Start believing the present circumstances and moving away from trusting God. Denial; flight; a change in what's important; how you spend your time, energy, and thoughts.)* Secrets; less time/energy for God, meetings, church; avoiding support and accountability people; superficial conversations; sarcasm; isolating; changes in goals; obsessed with relationships; breaking promises and commitments; neglecting family; preoccupation with material things, TV, computers, entertainment; procrastination; lying; overconfidence; bored; hiding money; image management; seeking to control situations and other people.

01. ______________________
______________________
02. ______________________
______________________
03. ______________________
______________________

## ANXIETY

*(Consumed by negative thoughts and undefined fear; getting energy from emotions.)* Worry, using profanity, being fearful; being resentful; replaying old, negative thoughts; perfectionism; judging other's motives; making goals and lists that you can't complete; mind reading; fantasy, codependent, rescuing; sleep problems, trouble concentrating, seeking/creating drama; gossip; using over-the-counter medication for pain, sleep or weight control; flirting.

01. ______

02. ______

03. ______

## SPEEDING UP

*(Trying to outrun the anxiety which is usually the first sign of depression.)* Super busy and always in a hurry (finding good reason to justify the work); workaholic; can't relax; avoiding slowing down; feeling driven; can't turn off thoughts; skipping meals; binge eating (usually at night); overspending; can't identify own feelings/needs; repetitive negative thoughts; irritable; dramatic mood swings; too much caffeine; over exercising; nervousness; difficulty being alone and/or with people; difficulty listening to others; making excuses for having to "do it all."

01. ______

02. ______

03. ______

## TICKED OFF

*(Getting adrenaline high on anger and aggression.)* Procrastination causing crisis in money, work, and relationships; increased sarcasm; black and white (all or nothing) thinking; feeling alone; nobody understands; overreacting, road rage; constant resentments; pushing others away; increasing isolation; blaming; arguing; irrational thinking; can't take criticism; defensive; people avoiding you; needing to be right; digestive problems; headaches; obsessive (stuck) thoughts; can't forgive; feeling superior; using intimidation.

01. ______________________________

______________________________

02. ______________________________

______________________________

03. ______________________________

______________________________

## EXHAUSTED

*(Loss of physical and emotional energy; coming off the adrenaline high, and the onset of depression.)* Depressed; panicked; confused; hopelessness; sleeping too much or too little; can't cope; overwhelmed; crying for "no reason"; can't think; forgetful; pessimistic; helpless; tired; numb; wanting to run; constant cravings for old coping behaviors; thinking of using sex, drugs, or alcohol; seeking old unhealthy people and places; really isolating; people angry with you; self abuse; suicidal thoughts; spontaneous crying; no goals; survival mode; not returning phone calls; missing work; irritability; no appetite.

01. ______________________________

______________________________

02. ______________________________

______________________________

03. ______________________________

______________________________

## RELAPSE

*(Returning to the place you swore you would never go again. Coping with life on your terms. You sitting in the driver's seat instead of God.)* Giving up and giving in; out of control; lost in your addiction; lying to yourself and others; feeling you just can't manage without your coping behaviors, at least for now. The result is the reinforcement of shame, guilt and condemnation; and feelings of abandonment and being alone.

01. ______________________________

______________________________

02. ______________________________

______________________________

03. ______________________________

______________________________

# Commitment To Change

Complete the Commitment to Change prior to your next group meeting.

Keep in mind, your Commitment to Change is often directly connected to the lowest level reached on the FASTER Scale. Healing happens best when we are fully aware of the challenges we face and take proactive steps to create change.

## LET'S PLAN FOR NEXT WEEK

### Commitment to change: what area do you need to change or what challenge are you facing this week?

- Double bind: what will it cost you if you change? If you don't change?
- How does this potential for change make you feel?
- What is your plan to maintain restoration regarding these changes?

### Who will you share your commitment with this week?

### What are the details of your accountability? What questions should they ask you?

BE PREPARED TO SHARE YOUR ANSWERS IN THIS CHAPTER WITH THE GUYS IN YOUR GROUP.

CHAPTER 12

# THE SUPERHERO ODYSSEY—PART 2

## Group Check-In

Complete the Group Check-In 24 hours before group.

### HOW DID YOU DO LAST WEEK?

01. How did you do on your Commitment to Change? ____________________

02. Did you lie directly or indirectly to anyone? ____________________

03. What did you do to improve significant relationships with your wife, family, or friends? ____________________

### WHERE ARE YOU RIGHT NOW?

04. What is the lowest level you identify with on the FASTER Scale? ____________________

# Diminishing Shame

As we learned this week, shame can sometimes serve as a Threshold Guardian, standing in the way of our continued growth, ability to change, and pursuit of healthy relationships.

Many people confuse shame with guilt or use these terms interchangeably. But they are really quite different.

**Guilt** is often defined as a feeling of having done something wrong or failed in an obligation. The focus is on the behavior: "I did something bad."

**Shame**, on the other hand, encompasses a spectrum of feelings—pain, humiliation, distress, worthlessness, disgrace, and more—and is not based on the person's behavior. The focus is on the person themselves: "I am something bad."

Many of us have experienced pain and trauma that resulted in a specific shame message: something we thought about ourselves based on what happened to us and how it made us feel. We then carry these shame messages with us in our heads; which serve as further proof that we are bad and reinforce that what we think about ourselves is true.

Shame-fueled messages sound like this:

- I'm not worthy of love and affection.
- I don't expect my needs to be met.
- When things go wrong, it's my fault.
- I will never be good enough.
- Taking risks will only hurt me.
- I'm a disappointment to my family.
- I don't deserve good things in my life.
- Being invisible keeps me safe.
- I'll never be as good as ______________________ (fill in a person's name).

When we carry shame-fueled messages like these, they become the filter by which we process all our experiences. To some extent, if all our experiences are filtered through these negative messages, then every experience—good or bad—will be tainted.

Getting rid of these shame-fueled messages is a crucial part of moving beyond this Threshold Guardian. Raising awareness of the messages we carry is the first step.

In the space below, identify any shame-fueled messages you carry. Then briefly explain where you think this message comes from: what experience created this message?

| SHAME-FUELED MESSAGE: | THIS MESSAGE COMES FROM: |
| --- | --- |
| | |
| | |
| | |
| | |
| | |

But we don't want to stop here. In order to keep moving forward as a Compassionate Warrior, we need to do what Jesus did:

> *...let us strip off every weight that slows us down, especially the sin that so easily trips us up. And let us run with endurance the race God has set before us. We do this by keeping our eyes on Jesus, the champion who initiates and perfects our faith.* ***Because of the joy awaiting him, he endured the cross, disregarding its shame.*** *Now he is seated in the place of honor beside God's throne.*
>
> HEBREWS 12:1-2 (NLT)

Although Jesus endured the shame of the Cross, He could easily disregard it—cast it out of His thoughts—because it was nothing compared to the glorious reward of spending eternity with God in heaven.[25]

The more we focus on who we are in Christ, the easier it will be for us to disregard the shame-fueled messages we carry and replace them with God-fueled messages that reflect who we are in Christ and the man God is calling us to be. (Some of your God-fueled messages could be the same as your personal/prophetic promises.)

For each shame-fueled message you identified, write a God-fueled message about who God says you are and/or is calling you to be.

Becoming a Compassionate Warrior is a one-day-at-a-time process. Each day, choosing to leave behind our old life and pursue the extraordinary life God has for us. Choose this today.

[25] Hebrews 12:2, Matthew Poole's Commentary, Bible Hub, https://biblehub.com/commentaries/hebrews/12-2.htm.

# FASTER Scale

Circle the behaviors on the FASTER Scale that you identify with in each section.
Identify the most powerful behavior in each section and write it next to the corresponding heading.
Answer the following three questions based on your most powerful or frequent behavior.

01. How does it affect me? How do I feel in the moment?
02. How does it affect the important people in my life?
03. Why do I do this? What is the benefit for me?

## RESTORATION ____________________

*(Accepting life on God's terms, with trust, grace, mercy, vulnerability and gratitude.)* No current secrets; working to resolve problems; identifying fears and feelings; keeping commitments to meetings, prayer, family, church, people, goals, and self; being open and honest, making eye contact; increasing in relationships with God and others; true accountability.

01. ____________________
02. ____________________
03. ____________________

## FORGETTING PRIORITIES ____________________

*(Start believing the present circumstances and moving away from trusting God. Denial; flight; a change in what's important; how you spend your time, energy, and thoughts.)* Secrets; less time/energy for God, meetings, church; avoiding support and accountability people; superficial conversations; sarcasm; isolating; changes in goals; obsessed with relationships; breaking promises and commitments; neglecting family; preoccupation with material things, TV, computers, entertainment; procrastination; lying; overconfidence; bored; hiding money; image management; seeking to control situations and other people.

01. ____________________
____________________
02. ____________________
____________________
03. ____________________
____________________

## ANXIETY

*(Consumed by negative thoughts and undefined fear; getting energy from emotions.)* Worry, using profanity, being fearful; being resentful; replaying old, negative thoughts; perfectionism; judging other's motives; making goals and lists that you can't complete; mind reading; fantasy, codependent, rescuing; sleep problems, trouble concentrating, seeking/creating drama; gossip; using over-the-counter medication for pain, sleep or weight control; flirting.

01. ______________________________

02. ______________________________

03. ______________________________

## SPEEDING UP

*(Trying to outrun the anxiety which is usually the first sign of depression.)* Super busy and always in a hurry (finding good reason to justify the work); workaholic; can't relax; avoiding slowing down; feeling driven; can't turn off thoughts; skipping meals; binge eating (usually at night); overspending; can't identify own feelings/needs; repetitive negative thoughts; irritable; dramatic mood swings; too much caffeine; over exercising; nervousness; difficulty being alone and/or with people; difficulty listening to others; making excuses for having to "do it all."

01. ______________________________

02. ______________________________

03. ______________________________

## TICKED OFF

*(Getting adrenaline high on anger and aggression.)* Procrastination causing crisis in money, work, and relationships; increased sarcasm; black and white (all or nothing) thinking; feeling alone; nobody understands; overreacting, road rage; constant resentments; pushing others away; increasing isolation; blaming; arguing; irrational thinking; can't take criticism; defensive; people avoiding you; needing to be right; digestive problems; headaches; obsessive (stuck) thoughts; can't forgive; feeling superior; using intimidation.

01. ______________________________________________

______________________________________________

02. ______________________________________________

______________________________________________

03. ______________________________________________

______________________________________________

## EXHAUSTED

*(Loss of physical and emotional energy; coming off the adrenaline high, and the onset of depression.)* Depressed; panicked; confused; hopelessness; sleeping too much or too little; can't cope; overwhelmed; crying for "no reason"; can't think; forgetful; pessimistic; helpless; tired; numb; wanting to run; constant cravings for old coping behaviors; thinking of using sex, drugs, or alcohol; seeking old unhealthy people and places; really isolating; people angry with you; self abuse; suicidal thoughts; spontaneous crying; no goals; survival mode; not returning phone calls; missing work; irritability; no appetite.

01. ______________________________________________

______________________________________________

02. ______________________________________________

______________________________________________

03. ______________________________________________

______________________________________________

## RELAPSE

*(Returning to the place you swore you would never go again. Coping with life on your terms. You sitting in the driver's seat instead of God.)* Giving up and giving in; out of control; lost in your addiction; lying to yourself and others; feeling you just can't manage without your coping behaviors, at least for now. The result is the reinforcement of shame, guilt and condemnation; and feelings of abandonment and being alone.

01. ______________________________________________

______________________________________________

02. ______________________________________________

______________________________________________

03. ______________________________________________

______________________________________________

# Commitment To Change

Complete the Commitment to Change prior to your next group meeting.

Keep in mind, your Commitment to Change is often directly connected to the lowest level reached on the FASTER Scale. Healing happens best when we are fully aware of the challenges we face and take proactive steps to create change.

## LET'S PLAN FOR NEXT WEEK

### Commitment to change: what area do you need to change or what challenge are you facing this week?

- Double bind: what will it cost you if you change? If you don't change?
- How does this potential for change make you feel?
- What is your plan to maintain restoration regarding these changes?

### Who will you share your commitment with this week?

### What are the details of your accountability? What questions should they ask you?

### BE PREPARED TO SHARE YOUR ANSWERS IN THIS CHAPTER WITH THE GUYS IN YOUR GROUP.

STAGE V

# WRAP UP

## What do you think?

You've come so far and are making great strides in your healing! What was the most life-changing thing you learned about yourself in Stage V? How is God using this to prepare you to help others?

# Progress, not Perfection

Becoming a Compassionate Warrior requires you to be brave. To take risks. To expand your world view and open up yourself to the amazing ways God is going to use you in the lives of others. What small steps are you taking that reflect progress in your healing journey?

| ISSUE | PERFECTION | WHERE I STARTED | PROGRESS |
|---|---|---|---|
| | | | |

What can you do this week to make progress toward your goal?

| ISSUE | PERFECTION | WHERE I STARTED | PROGRESS |
|---|---|---|---|
| | | | |

What can you do this week to make progress toward your goal?

| ISSUE | PERFECTION | WHERE I STARTED | PROGRESS |
| --- | --- | --- | --- |
| | | | |

What can you do this week to make progress toward your goal?

## Thoughts & Feelings Awareness Log

As we continue to learn what the life of a Compassionate Warrior looks like, we have to be cognizant of our emotions. With emotional self-awareness, we become skilled at managing our emotions—no longer allowing our emotions to control us or get the best of us. Recognizing and identifying your thoughts and feelings is a huge step in this process.

| I FELT... | ...BECAUSE I THOUGHT... |
| --- | --- |
| | |
| | |
| | |

The journaling and tools in this wrap up are for you, so you can evaluate what you're learning and keep track of the progress you're making. You don't have to share any of this with the guys in your group, but can if you want to.

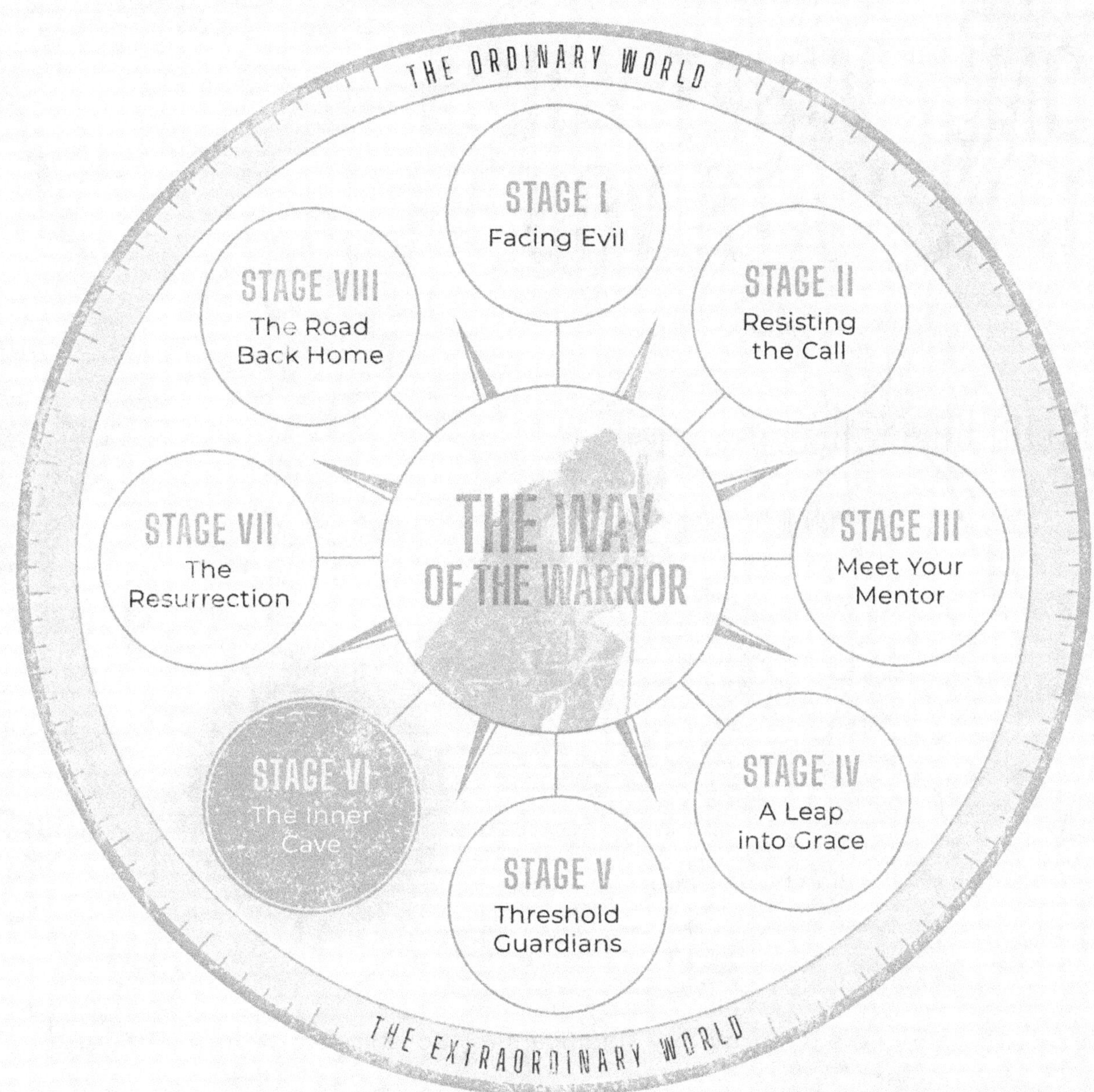


# STAGE VI

## THE INNER CAVE

CHAPTER 13

# ONLY WHAT YOU TAKE WITH YOU

## Group Check-In

Complete the Group Check-In 24 hours before group.

### HOW DID YOU DO LAST WEEK?

01. How did you do on your Commitment to Change? ______________________
______________________
______________________
______________________

02. Did you lie directly or indirectly to anyone? ______________________
______________________
______________________

03. What did you do to improve significant relationships with your wife, family, or friends? ______________________
______________________
______________________

### WHERE ARE YOU RIGHT NOW?

04. What is the lowest level you identify with on the FASTER Scale? ______________________
______________________
______________________

# Challenge Negative Thoughts

We all want to live out God's calling and purpose in our lives. But one thing that can interfere with this is being consumed by negative thoughts. Learning to navigate this requires us to be aware of when our negative thoughts begin to take over and also the strategies we need in place to challenge our negative thoughts.

Much of this journey happens in our mind. When we become better at identifying our negative thoughts, we can create positive thoughts that not only override our negative thoughts but bring life and health to the way we think about ourselves and others. One of the best ways to immediately counteract a negative thought is with a rational thought; a thought that is based on facts, logic, and reason, not based on how we feel.[26]

We can work to challenge and change our negative thoughts through practicing a rational response. This is how we learn to take healthy control of our thoughts.

> *For the weapons of our warfare are not of the flesh but have divine power to destroy strongholds. 5 We destroy arguments and every lofty opinion raised against the knowledge of God, and take every thought captive to obey Christ...*
>
> 2 CORINTHIANS 10:4-5 (ESV)

**Use the following table to identify a negative thought that continually takes up brain space and a rational thought that counteracts the negative thought.** Keep in mind: our negative thoughts create a lot of internal pressure for us. The goal of using rational thoughts is to take the pressure off of us and provide an alternative thought that is reasonable and freeing. Some examples are given to get you started.

| NEGATIVE THOUGHT | RATIONAL THOUGHT |
|---|---|
| *I'm not going to get the promotion because I'm not smart enough.* | *I'm smart enough to get this far in my job and to get the promotion—if I don't get this promotion, I know God has something better for me.* |
| *I will always be the needy little boy my mother said I am.* | *I'm not needy; having needs is a realistic human behavior. My mother's perception of me was based on her untreated pain and trauma. It was not about me.* |

26 Jeff Riggenbach, *The CBT Toolbox: A Workbook for Clients and Clinicians* (Eau Claire: Premier Publishing and Media, 2013), 54.

| NEGATIVE THOUGHT | RATIONAL THOUGHT |
|---|---|
| *Honesty and truth are overrated. The only way my marriage will last is by pretending to be the person she needs and hiding everything else.* | *Honesty and truth are the foundation of a healthy relationship. If I expect my wife to be her real, transparent self, I need to do the same.* |
| | |
| | |
| | |
| | |
| | |

Challenging our negative thoughts is part of the lifelong process of renewing the mind. Taking our thoughts captive and turning our focus toward God and His Word will help to dismantle the power these negative thoughts have over us.

# FASTER Scale

Circle the behaviors on the FASTER Scale that you identify with in each section.
Identify the most powerful behavior in each section and write it next to the corresponding heading.
Answer the following three questions based on your most powerful or frequent behavior.

01. How does it affect me? How do I feel in the moment?
02. How does it affect the important people in my life?
03. Why do I do this? What is the benefit for me?

## RESTORATION ______________________

*(Accepting life on God's terms, with trust, grace, mercy, vulnerability and gratitude.)* No current secrets; working to resolve problems; identifying fears and feelings; keeping commitments to meetings, prayer, family, church, people, goals, and self; being open and honest, making eye contact; increasing in relationships with God and others; true accountability.

01. ______________________
02. ______________________
03. ______________________

## FORGETTING PRIORITIES ______________________

*(Start believing the present circumstances and moving away from trusting God. Denial; flight; a change in what's important; how you spend your time, energy, and thoughts.)* Secrets; less time/energy for God, meetings, church; avoiding support and accountability people; superficial conversations; sarcasm; isolating; changes in goals; obsessed with relationships; breaking promises and commitments; neglecting family; preoccupation with material things, TV, computers, entertainment; procrastination; lying; overconfidence; bored; hiding money; image management; seeking to control situations and other people.

01. ______________________
______________________
02. ______________________
______________________
03. ______________________
______________________

## ANXIETY

*(Consumed by negative thoughts and undefined fear; getting energy from emotions.)* Worry, using profanity, being fearful; being resentful; replaying old, negative thoughts; perfectionism; judging other's motives; making goals and lists that you can't complete; mind reading; fantasy, codependent, rescuing; sleep problems, trouble concentrating, seeking/creating drama; gossip; using over-the-counter medication for pain, sleep or weight control; flirting.

01. ______

02. ______

03. ______

## SPEEDING UP

*(Trying to outrun the anxiety which is usually the first sign of depression.)* Super busy and always in a hurry (finding good reason to justify the work); workaholic; can't relax; avoiding slowing down; feeling driven; can't turn off thoughts; skipping meals; binge eating (usually at night); overspending; can't identify own feelings/needs; repetitive negative thoughts; irritable; dramatic mood swings; too much caffeine; over exercising; nervousness; difficulty being alone and/or with people; difficulty listening to others; making excuses for having to "do it all."

01. ______

02. ______

03. ______

## TICKED OFF

*(Getting adrenaline high on anger and aggression.)* Procrastination causing crisis in money, work, and relationships; increased sarcasm; black and white (all or nothing) thinking; feeling alone; nobody understands; overreacting, road rage; constant resentments; pushing others away; increasing isolation; blaming; arguing; irrational thinking; can't take criticism; defensive; people avoiding you; needing to be right; digestive problems; headaches; obsessive (stuck) thoughts; can't forgive; feeling superior; using intimidation.

01. ______________________________________________

______________________________________________

02. ______________________________________________

______________________________________________

03. ______________________________________________

______________________________________________

## EXHAUSTED ______________________________________________

*(Loss of physical and emotional energy; coming off the adrenaline high, and the onset of depression.)* Depressed; panicked; confused; hopelessness; sleeping too much or too little; can't cope; overwhelmed; crying for "no reason"; can't think; forgetful; pessimistic; helpless; tired; numb; wanting to run; constant cravings for old coping behaviors; thinking of using sex, drugs, or alcohol; seeking old unhealthy people and places; really isolating; people angry with you; self abuse; suicidal thoughts; spontaneous crying; no goals; survival mode; not returning phone calls; missing work; irritability; no appetite.

01. ______________________________________________

______________________________________________

02. ______________________________________________

______________________________________________

03. ______________________________________________

______________________________________________

## RELAPSE ______________________________________________

*(Returning to the place you swore you would never go again. Coping with life on your terms. You sitting in the driver's seat instead of God.)* Giving up and giving in; out of control; lost in your addiction; lying to yourself and others; feeling you just can't manage without your coping behaviors, at least for now. The result is the reinforcement of shame, guilt and condemnation; and feelings of abandonment and being alone.

01. ______________________________________________

______________________________________________

02. ______________________________________________

______________________________________________

03. ______________________________________________

______________________________________________

# Commitment To Change

Complete the Commitment to Change prior to your next group meeting.

Keep in mind, your Commitment to Change is often directly connected to the lowest level reached on the FASTER Scale. Healing happens best when we are fully aware of the challenges we face and take proactive steps to create change.

## LET'S PLAN FOR NEXT WEEK

### Commitment to change: what area do you need to change or what challenge are you facing this week?

- Double bind: what will it cost you if you change? If you don't change?
- How does this potential for change make you feel?
- What is your plan to maintain restoration regarding these changes?

### Who will you share your commitment with this week?

### What are the details of your accountability? What questions should they ask you?

**BE PREPARED TO SHARE YOUR ANSWERS IN THIS CHAPTER WITH THE GUYS IN YOUR GROUP.**

CHAPTER 14

# THE EXILE WITHIN IS FINALLY HONORED

## Group Check-In

Complete the Group Check-In 24 hours before group.

### HOW DID YOU DO LAST WEEK?

01. How did you do on your Commitment to Change? ______________________

02. Did you lie directly or indirectly to anyone? ______________________

03. What did you do to improve significant relationships with your wife, family, or friends? ______________________

### WHERE ARE YOU RIGHT NOW?

04. What is the lowest level you identify with on the FASTER Scale? ______________________

# Internal Family Systems

Internal Family Systems (IFS) therapy was developed by Richard Schwartz as he worked with clients who struggled with eating disorders.[27] Curious about what motivated their behaviors, he conducted a series of interviews and was surprised by how patients described the different voices in their head that regularly participated in ongoing conversations. He describes it this way:

"The more I explored these questions, the more their descriptions felt familiar to me as a family therapist, as if I were interviewing one family member about the rest of her family. It seemed that each voice had a distinct character, complete with idiosyncratic desires, styles of communication, and temperaments, and that these voices interacted like conflicting parties in a family struggle: alternately protecting and distracting, allying and battling with each other."[28]

Within this model, used by Christian and secular therapists, the internal psychological system of every person is made up of several **Parts**.

In her book, *Altogether You*, Jenna Riemersma describes it this way:

> **Parts:** *Unique aspects of our personalities (subpersonalities) that have their own thoughts, feelings, sensations, and agendas. All people are born with many unburdened parts that together comprise their unique personality. All parts want something positive for the individual. Some parts become burdened with pain (or strategies for coping with pain) from negative life experiences.*[29]

The core **Self** is at the center of this internal system, which "...holds and expresses the compassion, courage, curiosity, clarity, confidence, creativity, calm, and ability to connect to others."[30] The Self reflects our basic human nature created by God that we were born with. All of us, to some extent, have experienced pain and trauma in our lives, which results in sadness, fear, shame, and emotional pain. This residual emotional pain is labeled **Exiles** in this model.

---

[27] Richard Schwartz, "Our Multiple Selves: Applying systems thinking to the inner family," *The Family Therapy Networker*, March-April edition, 1987.

[28] Richard Schwartz, *The Family Therapy Networker*, 1987.

[29] Jenna Riemersma, *Altogether You: Experiencing personal and spiritual transformation with Internal Family Systems therapy* (Marietta: Pivotal Press, 2020), 5.

[30] Arthur Mones and Richard Schwartz, "The Functional Hypothesis: A Family Systems Contribution Toward an Understanding of the Healing Process of the Common Factors," *Journal of Psychotherapy Integration, 17*(4), 2007, 322.

In order to compartmentalize and guard the Self from ever feeling painful Exiles, two other types of Parts are activated. One type is called **Managers**: they diligently work to control and keep things locked down, protecting the person from experiencing pain, but often creating other problems in the process. The other type is called **Firefighters**: their goal is the same, to protect from emotional pain; however, instead of being hypervigilant, they use tactics that sooth and distract from the pain, commonly taking the form of addictive behaviors.

There's a lot of information in this brief snapshot of IFS, so let's break it down.

We all have various **Parts** of ourselves that help to navigate our internal world.

- The **Self** is who we are at our core, who God originally created us to be.
- **Exiles** are the emotionally painful parts of ourselves we carry from past pain and trauma.
- **Managers** protect us *proactively* through control and hypervigilance (actually giving us a false sense of safety), helping us think we can avoid emotional pain.
- **Firefighters** protect us *reactively* through distraction, providing activities to medicate our pain so we don't feel it.

It might seem a bit strange to talk about these various aspects of ourselves as "Parts." But even the apostle Paul struggled with understanding his various parts:

> *For I do not understand my own actions. For I do not do what I want, but I do the very thing I hate.*
>
> ROMANS 7:15 (ESV)

And, as Jenna says,

> *...if the word part feels uncomfortable, replace it with a word like component, aspect, or subpersonality. The important insight is not what we call it, but the ability to realize that when I'm feeling or doing something I don't want to feel or do, I'm not a bad person, I simply have parts at war.*[31]

---

31 Jenna Riemersma, *Altogether You: Experiencing personal and spiritual transformation with Internal Family Systems therapy* (Marietta: Pivotal Press, 2020), 6.

Thinking about your own situation, where have you seen some of your managers and firefighters trying to help you avoid feeling the pain of your exiles? Use the following table to help you identify your managers, firefighters, and the way they're trying to help you.

| MANAGERS (PROACTIVE STRATEGIES): | ...TRYING TO HELP YOU AVOID FEELING... |
| --- | --- |
| | |
| | |
| | |
| | |

| MANAGERS (REACTIVE STRATEGIES): | ...TRYING TO HELP YOU AVOID FEELING... |
| --- | --- |
| | |
| | |
| | |
| | |

The more we can do to get to know these parts of ourselves—how they were created out of our pain and trauma, and how they're trying to protect us—the better equipped we are to make sense of our story.

# FASTER Scale

Circle the behaviors on the FASTER Scale that you identify with in each section.
Identify the most powerful behavior in each section and write it next to the corresponding heading.
Answer the following three questions based on your most powerful or frequent behavior.

01. How does it affect me? How do I feel in the moment?
02. How does it affect the important people in my life?
03. Why do I do this? What is the benefit for me?

## RESTORATION ______

*(Accepting life on God's terms, with trust, grace, mercy, vulnerability and gratitude.)* No current secrets; working to resolve problems; identifying fears and feelings; keeping commitments to meetings, prayer, family, church, people, goals, and self; being open and honest, making eye contact; increasing in relationships with God and others; true accountability.

01. ______
02. ______
03. ______

## FORGETTING PRIORITIES ______

*(Start believing the present circumstances and moving away from trusting God. Denial; flight; a change in what's important; how you spend your time, energy, and thoughts.)* Secrets; less time/energy for God, meetings, church; avoiding support and accountability people; superficial conversations; sarcasm; isolating; changes in goals; obsessed with relationships; breaking promises and commitments; neglecting family; preoccupation with material things, TV, computers, entertainment; procrastination; lying; overconfidence; bored; hiding money; image management; seeking to control situations and other people.

01. ______
02. ______
03. ______

## ANXIETY

*(Consumed by negative thoughts and undefined fear; getting energy from emotions.)* Worry, using profanity, being fearful; being resentful; replaying old, negative thoughts; perfectionism; judging other's motives; making goals and lists that you can't complete; mind reading; fantasy, codependent, rescuing; sleep problems, trouble concentrating, seeking/creating drama; gossip; using over-the-counter medication for pain, sleep or weight control; flirting.

01. ______________________________

02. ______________________________

03. ______________________________

## SPEEDING UP

*(Trying to outrun the anxiety which is usually the first sign of depression.)* Super busy and always in a hurry (finding good reason to justify the work); workaholic; can't relax; avoiding slowing down; feeling driven; can't turn off thoughts; skipping meals; binge eating (usually at night); overspending; can't identify own feelings/needs; repetitive negative thoughts; irritable; dramatic mood swings; too much caffeine; over exercising; nervousness; difficulty being alone and/or with people; difficulty listening to others; making excuses for having to "do it all."

01. ______________________________

02. ______________________________

03. ______________________________

## TICKED OFF

*(Getting adrenaline high on anger and aggression.)* Procrastination causing crisis in money, work, and relationships; increased sarcasm; black and white (all or nothing) thinking; feeling alone; nobody understands; overreacting, road rage; constant resentments; pushing others away; increasing isolation; blaming; arguing; irrational thinking; can't take criticism; defensive; people avoiding you; needing to be right; digestive problems; headaches; obsessive (stuck) thoughts; can't forgive; feeling superior; using intimidation.

01. ______________________________

______________________________

02. ______________________________

______________________________

03. ______________________________

______________________________

## EXHAUSTED ______________________________

*(Loss of physical and emotional energy; coming off the adrenaline high, and the onset of depression.)* Depressed; panicked; confused; hopelessness; sleeping too much or too little; can't cope; overwhelmed; crying for "no reason"; can't think; forgetful; pessimistic; helpless; tired; numb; wanting to run; constant cravings for old coping behaviors; thinking of using sex, drugs, or alcohol; seeking old unhealthy people and places; really isolating; people angry with you; self abuse; suicidal thoughts; spontaneous crying; no goals; survival mode; not returning phone calls; missing work; irritability; no appetite.

01. ______________________________

______________________________

02. ______________________________

______________________________

03. ______________________________

______________________________

## RELAPSE ______________________________

*(Returning to the place you swore you would never go again. Coping with life on your terms. You sitting in the driver's seat instead of God.)* Giving up and giving in; out of control; lost in your addiction; lying to yourself and others; feeling you just can't manage without your coping behaviors, at least for now. The result is the reinforcement of shame, guilt and condemnation; and feelings of abandonment and being alone.

01. ______________________________

______________________________

02. ______________________________

______________________________

03. ______________________________

______________________________

# Commitment To Change

Complete the Commitment to Change prior to your next group meeting.

Keep in mind, your Commitment to Change is often directly connected to the lowest level reached on the FASTER Scale. Healing happens best when we are fully aware of the challenges we face and take proactive steps to create change.

## LET'S PLAN FOR NEXT WEEK

### Commitment to change: what area do you need to change or what challenge are you facing this week?

- Double bind: what will it cost you if you change? If you don't change?
- How does this potential for change make you feel?
- What is your plan to maintain restoration regarding these changes?

### Who will you share your commitment with this week?

### What are the details of your accountability? What questions should they ask you?

BE PREPARED TO SHARE YOUR ANSWERS IN THIS CHAPTER WITH THE GUYS IN YOUR GROUP.

STAGE VI

# WRAP UP

## What do you think?

This journey will take you to the deepest parts of yourself, explore the ways you've conquered recovery, and reveal God's purpose in your life. Considering all you've learned through Stage VI of this journey, how is God revealing His purpose and plan for your life?

# Progress, not Perfection

Many of us tend to struggle with the same things over and over in our lives. This is especially true when it comes to our healing. Noticing progress in these challenging areas is crucial and may prove to be even more impactful because we see the changes happening. Even if it's small, the change—the progress—is noteworthy.

| ISSUE | PERFECTION | WHERE I STARTED | PROGRESS |
| --- | --- | --- | --- |
| | | | |

What can you do this week to make progress toward your goal?

| ISSUE | PERFECTION | WHERE I STARTED | PROGRESS |
| --- | --- | --- | --- |
| | | | |

What can you do this week to make progress toward your goal?

| ISSUE | PERFECTION | WHERE I STARTED | PROGRESS |
|---|---|---|---|
| | | | |

What can you do this week to make progress toward your goal?

## Thoughts & Feelings Awareness Log

Tracking our thoughts and feelings is tough work. At times, stuffing down or attempting to ignore our feelings seems like a better solution. But it's not. When we learn to connect our thoughts and feelings, and express them in a healthy way, it continues to move us toward life-changing health and wholeness.

| I FELT... | ...BECAUSE I THOUGHT... |
|---|---|
| | |
| | |
| | |

The journaling and tools in this wrap up are for you, so you can evaluate what you're learning and keep track of the progress you're making. You don't have to share any of this with the guys in your group, but can if you want to.

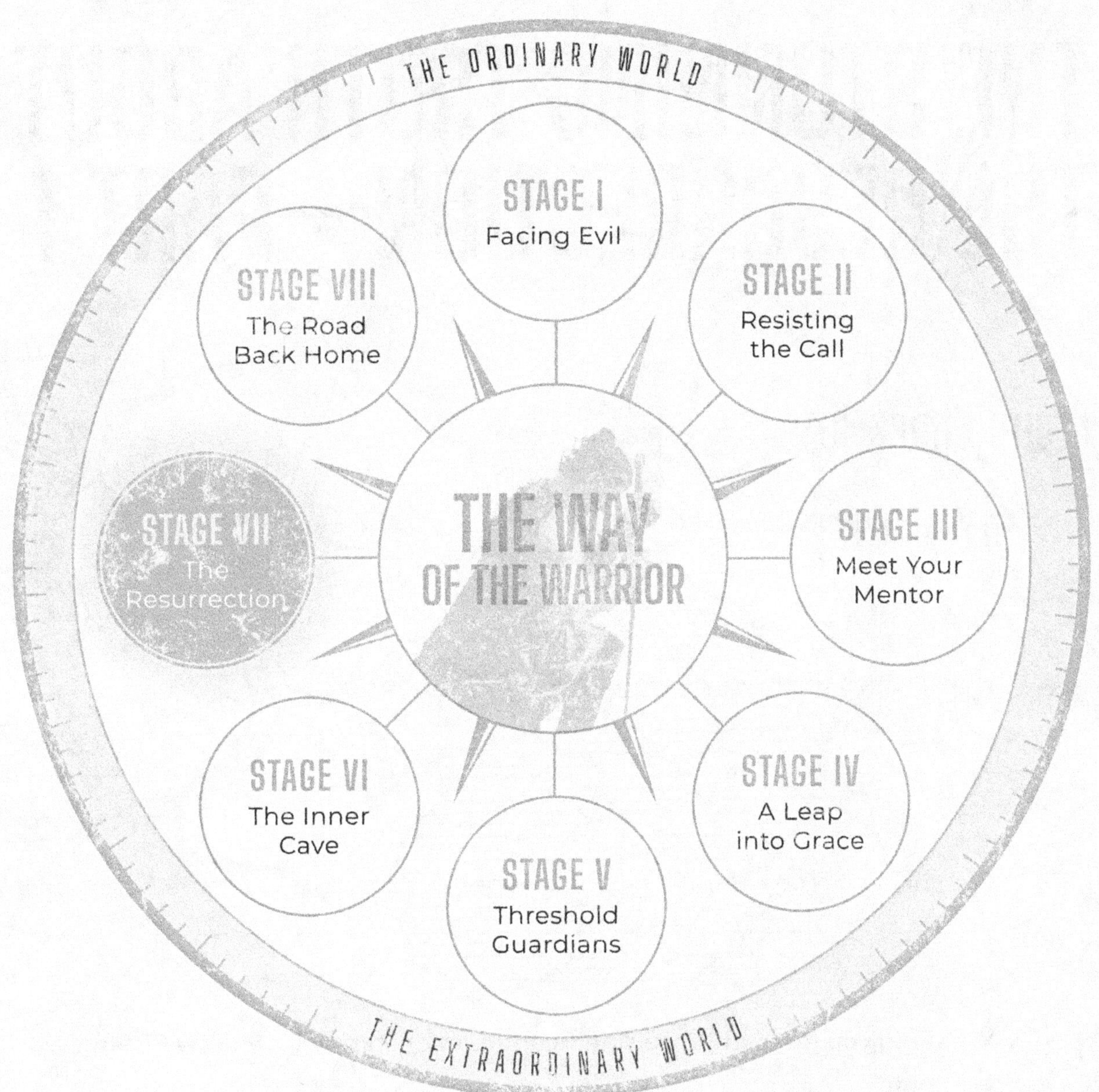


# STAGE VII

## THE RESURRECTION

# CHAPTER 15
# THE STUNNING TRUTH ABOUT THE RESURRECTION—PART 1

## Group Check-In

Complete the Group Check-In 24 hours before group.

### HOW DID YOU DO LAST WEEK?

01. How did you do on your Commitment to Change? ______________________________

____________________________________________________________

____________________________________________________________

____________________________________________________________

02. Did you lie directly or indirectly to anyone? ______________________________

____________________________________________________________

____________________________________________________________

03. What did you do to improve significant relationships with your wife, family, or friends? ______________________________

____________________________________________________________

____________________________________________________________

### WHERE ARE YOU RIGHT NOW?

04. What is the lowest level you identify with on the FASTER Scale? ______________

____________________________________________________________

____________________________________________________________

# The Power of Words

In the chapter this week, we talked about how our heart for God and His plan for us is often tested through the challenges we face in life. One of the greatest challenges for many men is relationships. We know God created us for relationships with Him and others. So why does this seem to be so difficult?

As previously mentioned, many men were never taught some key aspects of building relationships. Being able to recognize and understand our emotions, AND being able to communicate our feelings to another person, are huge when it comes to relationships.

Too often, when we lack emotional awareness, our feelings show up in unpredictable ways. We may not recognize how a situation is making us feel until we get caught up in our reaction and emotionally explode on the people around us. This is not helpful for us or our relationships.

Being able to use our words to communicate what we think and how we feel about a situation is foundational to cultivating healthy relationships. It's even more important when we consider what Scripture says about the power of our words.

> *A gentle answer turns away wrath, but a harsh word stirs up anger.*
>
> PROVERBS 15:1 (NIV)

> *The heart of the godly thinks carefully before speaking;...*
>
> PROVERBS 15:28 (NLT)

> *Kind words are like honey—sweet to the soul and healthy for the body.*
>
> PROVERBS 16:24 (NLT)

> *What you say can preserve life or destroy it; so you must accept the consequences of your words.*
>
> PROVERBS 18:21 (GNT)

> *Wise words are more valuable than much gold and many rubies.*
>
> PROVERBS 20:15 (NLT)

If we want to communicate our thoughts and feelings in a healthy way during any situation, it's going to take practice. Use the following space to walk through a few recent situations and practice communicating a healthy response.

First, describe a recent situation where you needed to communicate your thoughts and feelings. Second, describe how the situation actually turned out. Third, if you could do it over again, how would you communicate your thoughts and feelings in a way that would bring about a better resolution? If possible, use situations that involve different people (spouse, kids, a friend, a family member).

*Example*:

| **Situation:** *When I came home from work the other day, my wife and son were in an argument. My wife expected me to jump in and get involved without knowing much about the issue.* | **How it actually turned out:** *Feeling overwhelmed by my workday, I sarcastically said, "You guys started this without me. I'm sure you can figure it out." I walked away but ended up arguing with my wife about it later.* |
|---|---|
| **If I could do it over again:** *When I came home to the argument between my wife and son, I would say to my wife, "Babe, I've had a stressful day. Can I take a few minutes to get into a good headspace before jumping into this?" When returning to the room, I would say to my wife, "Will you please explain what's going on?" I would listen carefully and respectfully. I would ask my son, "Is there anything you would like to add to what your mother has said?" I would listen carefully and respectfully. Then I would say, "I can see how frustrated this is making both of you. I would be frustrated too. I think..." and then use my words to help bring about a good resolution.* | |

| **Situation:** | **How it actually turned out:** |
|---|---|
| **If I could do it over again:** | |

| Situation: | How it actually turned out: |
|---|---|
| If I could do it over again: | |

| Situation: | How it actually turned out: |
|---|---|
| If I could do it over again: | |

Learning how to communicate our thoughts and feelings is such a vital piece of our healing journey. When we are able to communicate well, even during difficult conversations, it brings life to the relationship; it shows others that we respect, value, and care about them. This is the power of words.

# FASTER Scale

Circle the behaviors on the FASTER Scale that you identify with in each section.
Identify the most powerful behavior in each section and write it next to the corresponding heading.
Answer the following three questions based on your most powerful or frequent behavior.

01. How does it affect me? How do I feel in the moment?
02. How does it affect the important people in my life?
03. Why do I do this? What is the benefit for me?

## RESTORATION ______________________________

*(Accepting life on God's terms, with trust, grace, mercy, vulnerability and gratitude.)* No current secrets; working to resolve problems; identifying fears and feelings; keeping commitments to meetings, prayer, family, church, people, goals, and self; being open and honest, making eye contact; increasing in relationships with God and others; true accountability.

01. ______________________________
02. ______________________________
03. ______________________________

## FORGETTING PRIORITIES ______________________________

*(Start believing the present circumstances and moving away from trusting God. Denial; flight; a change in what's important; how you spend your time, energy, and thoughts.)* Secrets; less time/energy for God, meetings, church; avoiding support and accountability people; superficial conversations; sarcasm; isolating; changes in goals; obsessed with relationships; breaking promises and commitments; neglecting family; preoccupation with material things, TV, computers, entertainment; procrastination; lying; overconfidence; bored; hiding money; image management; seeking to control situations and other people.

01. ______________________________
______________________________
02. ______________________________
______________________________
03. ______________________________
______________________________

## ANXIETY

*(Consumed by negative thoughts and undefined fear; getting energy from emotions.)* Worry, using profanity, being fearful; being resentful; replaying old, negative thoughts; perfectionism; judging other's motives; making goals and lists that you can't complete; mind reading; fantasy, codependent, rescuing; sleep problems, trouble concentrating, seeking/creating drama; gossip; using over-the-counter medication for pain, sleep or weight control; flirting.

01. ______________________________

02. ______________________________

03. ______________________________

## SPEEDING UP

*(Trying to outrun the anxiety which is usually the first sign of depression.)* Super busy and always in a hurry (finding good reason to justify the work); workaholic; can't relax; avoiding slowing down; feeling driven; can't turn off thoughts; skipping meals; binge eating (usually at night); overspending; can't identify own feelings/needs; repetitive negative thoughts; irritable; dramatic mood swings; too much caffeine; over exercising; nervousness; difficulty being alone and/or with people; difficulty listening to others; making excuses for having to "do it all."

01. ______________________________

02. ______________________________

03. ______________________________

## TICKED OFF

*(Getting adrenaline high on anger and aggression.)* Procrastination causing crisis in money, work, and relationships; increased sarcasm; black and white (all or nothing) thinking; feeling alone; nobody understands; overreacting, road rage; constant resentments; pushing others away; increasing isolation; blaming; arguing; irrational thinking; can't take criticism; defensive; people avoiding you; needing to be right; digestive problems; headaches; obsessive (stuck) thoughts; can't forgive; feeling superior; using intimidation.

01. ______________________________________________

______________________________________________

02. ______________________________________________

______________________________________________

03. ______________________________________________

______________________________________________

## EXHAUSTED

*(Loss of physical and emotional energy; coming off the adrenaline high, and the onset of depression.)* Depressed; panicked; confused; hopelessness; sleeping too much or too little; can't cope; overwhelmed; crying for "no reason"; can't think; forgetful; pessimistic; helpless; tired; numb; wanting to run; constant cravings for old coping behaviors; thinking of using sex, drugs, or alcohol; seeking old unhealthy people and places; really isolating; people angry with you; self abuse; suicidal thoughts; spontaneous crying; no goals; survival mode; not returning phone calls; missing work; irritability; no appetite.

01. ______________________________________________

______________________________________________

02. ______________________________________________

______________________________________________

03. ______________________________________________

______________________________________________

## RELAPSE

*(Returning to the place you swore you would never go again. Coping with life on your terms. You sitting in the driver's seat instead of God.)* Giving up and giving in; out of control; lost in your addiction; lying to yourself and others; feeling you just can't manage without your coping behaviors, at least for now. The result is the reinforcement of shame, guilt and condemnation; and feelings of abandonment and being alone.

01. ______________________________________________

______________________________________________

02. ______________________________________________

______________________________________________

03. ______________________________________________

______________________________________________

# Commitment To Change

Complete the Commitment to Change prior to your next group meeting.

Keep in mind, your Commitment to Change is often directly connected to the lowest level reached on the FASTER Scale. Healing happens best when we are fully aware of the challenges we face and take proactive steps to create change.

## LET'S PLAN FOR NEXT WEEK

Commitment to change: what area do you need to change or what challenge are you facing this week?

- Double bind: what will it cost you if you change? If you don't change?
- How does this potential for change make you feel?
- What is your plan to maintain restoration regarding these changes?

Who will you share your commitment with this week?

What are the details of your accountability? What questions should they ask you?

BE PREPARED TO SHARE YOUR ANSWERS IN THIS CHAPTER WITH THE GUYS IN YOUR GROUP.

CHAPTER 16

# THE STUNNING TRUTH ABOUT THE RESURRECTION—PART 2

## Group Check-In

Complete the Group Check-In 24 hours before group.

### HOW DID YOU DO LAST WEEK?

01. How did you do on your Commitment to Change? ______

02. Did you lie directly or indirectly to anyone? ______

03. What did you do to improve significant relationships with your wife, family, or friends? ______

### WHERE ARE YOU RIGHT NOW?

04. What is the lowest level you identify with on the FASTER Scale? ______

# Developing Empathy

This process of changing and growing into a Compassionate Warrior has required us to learn about ourselves and see ourselves differently; to see ourselves the way God sees us. The more we get to know God and who He is, the easier it is to see ourselves—our God-given qualities and characteristics—through His eyes and gain a healthy perspective of who God created us to be. This is what happens when we invest in the relationship we have with our heavenly Father.

As we get healthier, we begin to recognize ways we can invest in our other important relationships. Over time, we become empathetic toward others. This equips us to understand and appreciate the qualities and characteristics God has given our wife; the unique way God made her that will help her become the woman He created her to be.

> In the alphabetized list below, identify a quality, characteristic, or skill your wife possesses that you recognize and appreciate about her (at least one for each letter).[32] If you are not married and hope to be some day, complete this exercise based on the qualities and characteristics you would like in a future wife. It's okay if you can't get all 26 letters, but take time to fill in as many as you can!

*Examples: E - encouraging; H - humble; M - makes birthdays/holidays special; P - patient; T - tends to the elderly in our church; Y - yields to God's leading in her life.*

**My wife (is)...**

- A ______________________
- B ______________________
- C ______________________
- D ______________________
- E ______________________
- F ______________________
- G ______________________
- H ______________________
- I ______________________
- J ______________________
- K ______________________
- L ______________________
- M ______________________
- N ______________________
- O ______________________
- P ______________________
- Q ______________________
- R ______________________
- S ______________________
- T ______________________
- U ______________________
- V ______________________
- W ______________________
- X ______________________
- Y ______________________
- Z ______________________

[32] Jeff Riggenbach, *The CBT Toolbox: A Workbook for Clients and Clinicians* (Eau Claire: Premier Publishing and Media, 2013), 34.

Which one or two of these could you praise your wife for this week? How will you make this happen?

**Note:** *Help Her Heal: An Empathy Workbook for Sex Addicts to Help their Partners Heal* is a great resource for developing empathy and healing broken relationships.

Write a prayer for your wife, asking God to give her the strength and courage she needs to become the woman He created her to be. (If you're not married, and hope to be some day, write a prayer for your future wife.)

Write a prayer for yourself, asking God to give you the strength and courage you need to become the man He created you to be.

Developing empathy happens over time, as we become more compassionate and learn to feel what others are feeling, as though we're experiencing it ourselves. This changes us and is a key component to transforming relationships.

# FASTER Scale

Circle the behaviors on the FASTER Scale that you identify with in each section.
Identify the most powerful behavior in each section and write it next to the corresponding heading.
Answer the following three questions based on your most powerful or frequent behavior.

01. How does it affect me? How do I feel in the moment?
02. How does it affect the important people in my life?
03. Why do I do this? What is the benefit for me?

## RESTORATION ____________________

*(Accepting life on God's terms, with trust, grace, mercy, vulnerability and gratitude.)* No current secrets; working to resolve problems; identifying fears and feelings; keeping commitments to meetings, prayer, family, church, people, goals, and self; being open and honest, making eye contact; increasing in relationships with God and others; true accountability.

01. ____________________
02. ____________________
03. ____________________

## FORGETTING PRIORITIES ____________________

*(Start believing the present circumstances and moving away from trusting God. Denial; flight; a change in what's important; how you spend your time, energy, and thoughts.)* Secrets; less time/energy for God, meetings, church; avoiding support and accountability people; superficial conversations; sarcasm; isolating; changes in goals; obsessed with relationships; breaking promises and commitments; neglecting family; preoccupation with material things, TV, computers, entertainment; procrastination; lying; overconfidence; bored; hiding money; image management; seeking to control situations and other people.

01. ____________________
____________________
02. ____________________
____________________
03. ____________________
____________________

## ANXIETY

*(Consumed by negative thoughts and undefined fear; getting energy from emotions.)* Worry, using profanity, being fearful; being resentful; replaying old, negative thoughts; perfectionism; judging other's motives; making goals and lists that you can't complete; mind reading; fantasy, codependent, rescuing; sleep problems, trouble concentrating, seeking/creating drama; gossip; using over-the-counter medication for pain, sleep or weight control; flirting.

01. ______________________________

02. ______________________________

03. ______________________________

## SPEEDING UP

*(Trying to outrun the anxiety which is usually the first sign of depression.)* Super busy and always in a hurry (finding good reason to justify the work); workaholic; can't relax; avoiding slowing down; feeling driven; can't turn off thoughts; skipping meals; binge eating (usually at night); overspending; can't identify own feelings/needs; repetitive negative thoughts; irritable; dramatic mood swings; too much caffeine; over exercising; nervousness; difficulty being alone and/or with people; difficulty listening to others; making excuses for having to "do it all."

01. ______________________________

02. ______________________________

03. ______________________________

## TICKED OFF

*(Getting adrenaline high on anger and aggression.)* Procrastination causing crisis in money, work, and relationships; increased sarcasm; black and white (all or nothing) thinking; feeling alone; nobody understands; overreacting, road rage; constant resentments; pushing others away; increasing isolation; blaming; arguing; irrational thinking; can't take criticism; defensive; people avoiding you; needing to be right; digestive problems; headaches; obsessive (stuck) thoughts; can't forgive; feeling superior; using intimidation.

01. ______________________________

02. ______________________________

03. ______________________________

## EXHAUSTED ______________________________

*(Loss of physical and emotional energy; coming off the adrenaline high, and the onset of depression.)* Depressed; panicked; confused; hopelessness; sleeping too much or too little; can't cope; overwhelmed; crying for "no reason"; can't think; forgetful; pessimistic; helpless; tired; numb; wanting to run; constant cravings for old coping behaviors; thinking of using sex, drugs, or alcohol; seeking old unhealthy people and places; really isolating; people angry with you; self abuse; suicidal thoughts; spontaneous crying; no goals; survival mode; not returning phone calls; missing work; irritability; no appetite.

01. ______________________________

02. ______________________________

03. ______________________________

## RELAPSE ______________________________

*(Returning to the place you swore you would never go again. Coping with life on your terms. You sitting in the driver's seat instead of God.)* Giving up and giving in; out of control; lost in your addiction; lying to yourself and others; feeling you just can't manage without your coping behaviors, at least for now. The result is the reinforcement of shame, guilt and condemnation; and feelings of abandonment and being alone.

01. ______________________________

02. ______________________________

03. ______________________________

# Commitment To Change

Complete the Commitment to Change prior to your next group meeting.

Keep in mind, your Commitment to Change is often directly connected to the lowest level reached on the FASTER Scale. Healing happens best when we are fully aware of the challenges we face and take proactive steps to create change.

## LET'S PLAN FOR NEXT WEEK

### Commitment to change: what area do you need to change or what challenge are you facing this week?

- Double bind: what will it cost you if you change? If you don't change?
- How does this potential for change make you feel?
- What is your plan to maintain restoration regarding these changes?

### Who will you share your commitment with this week?

### What are the details of your accountability? What questions should they ask you?

BE PREPARED TO SHARE YOUR ANSWERS IN THIS CHAPTER WITH THE GUYS IN YOUR GROUP.

STAGE VII

# WRAP UP

## What do you think?

> The work you're doing is life-changing; not only for you but for those around you. Healing is contagious! As you spend time journaling, focus on ways you've seen changes in those around you because of your healing. Pay attention to their behaviors and the words they use. Does it reflect the behaviors and words you're learning through this healing journey?

# Progress, not Perfection

This journey is not only for a few months or for a season; it's a lifelong journey. The small incremental steps you take that show progress accumulate over time. They give you hope. They help you to be more in tune and focused on areas you want to improve. They help you to thrive! What areas are you noticing progress in helping you become a Compassionate Warrior?

| ISSUE | PERFECTION | WHERE I STARTED | PROGRESS |
|---|---|---|---|
| | | | |

What can you do this week to make progress toward your goal?

| ISSUE | PERFECTION | WHERE I STARTED | PROGRESS |
|---|---|---|---|
| | | | |

What can you do this week to make progress toward your goal?

| ISSUE | PERFECTION | WHERE I STARTED | PROGRESS |
|---|---|---|---|
| | | | |

What can you do this week to make progress toward your goal?

## Thoughts & Feelings Awareness Log

Even when making great strides in our healing, sometimes our feelings of shame, worthlessness, and fear take over and create chaos in our thought processes. When this happens, take control of your negative thoughts by replacing them with positive thoughts and watch your feelings follow.

| I FELT... | ...BECAUSE I THOUGHT... |
|---|---|
| | |
| | |
| | |

The journaling and tools in this wrap up are for you, so you can evaluate what you're learning and keep track of the progress you're making. You don't have to share any of this with the guys in your group, but can if you want to.

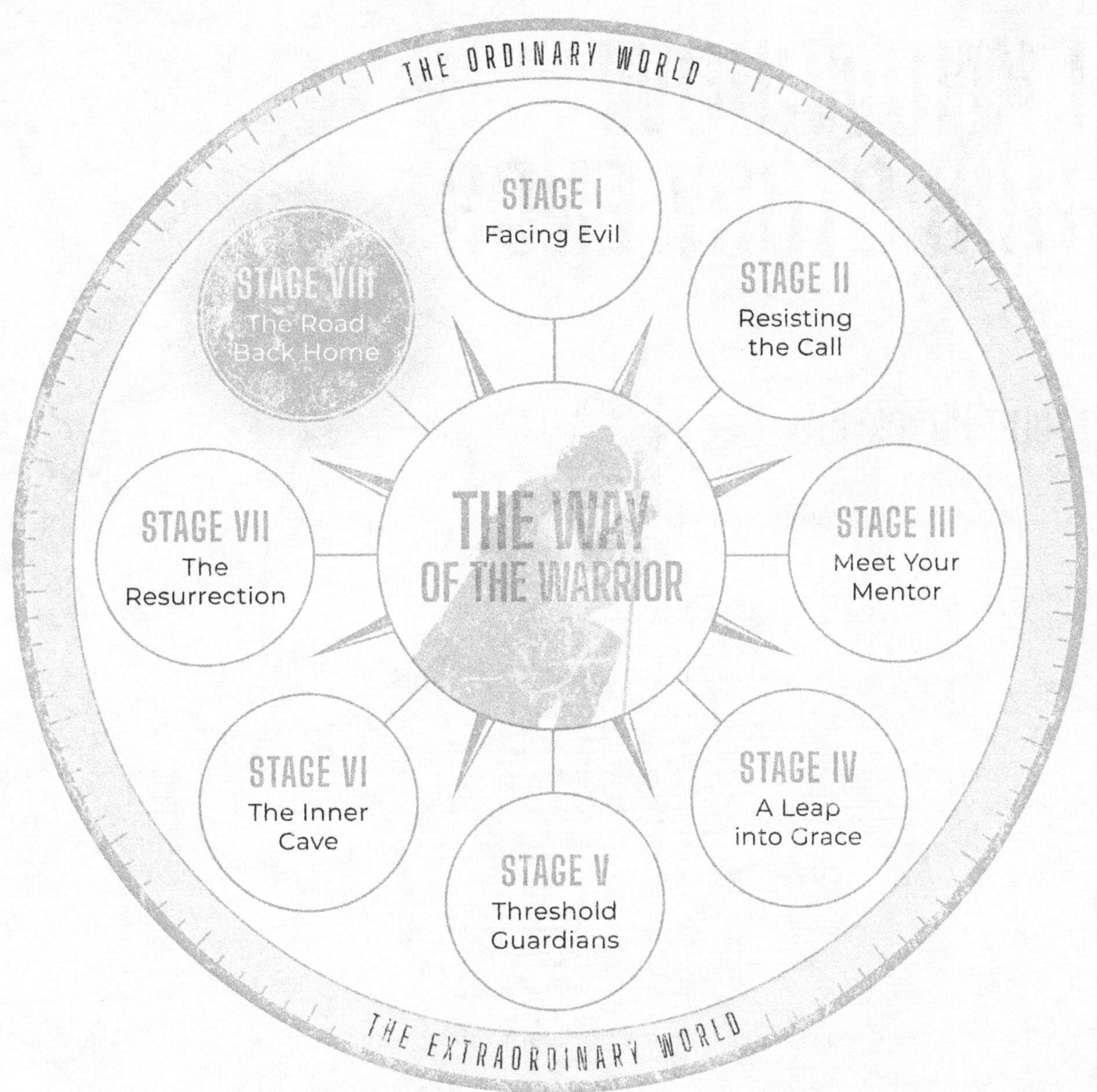


# STAGE VIII

## THE ROAD BACK HOME

CHAPTER 17

# I KNOW HOW THIS STORY ENDS

## Group Check-In

Complete the Group Check-In 24 hours before group.

### HOW DID YOU DO LAST WEEK?

01. How did you do on your Commitment to Change? ____________________

02. Did you lie directly or indirectly to anyone? ____________________

03. What did you do to improve significant relationships with your wife, family, or friends? ____________________

### WHERE ARE YOU RIGHT NOW?

04. What is the lowest level you identify with on the FASTER Scale? ____________________

# Developing Positive Self-Talk

As we've learned, the Hero's Journey focuses on answering a call on our lives—to no longer be content with the ordinary or areas of unhealth, but motivated to change so we can live the extraordinary life God has for us.

In the movie, *What About Bob?*,[33] Bob Wiley has a mantra he says over and over to calm himself, in an attempt to reduce his anxiety: "I feel good. I feel great. I feel wonderful." But you can tell by the expression on his face that he doesn't really believe what he was saying to himself.

Even if we repeat our mantra over and over, if we don't believe what we're saying, it won't help to calm the voice of our inner critic. And it needs to be grounded in God's Word to bring about lasting change. This is what makes self-talk so important. When we are pursuing lifelong health and healing, we need to make sure that what we're saying to ourselves is compassionate and caring. We need to talk to ourselves the same way we would talk to a friend or loved one who is hurting. Developing positive self-talk takes time and practice, and can make a significant difference in creating a mindset for healing.

In the following table, write out a few things you like about yourself or characteristics you're developing in yourself. As you think about what you like about yourself or are developing in yourself, identify how it makes you feel. Then, add a Scripture that reinforces this identity you see in yourself. (If you need help finding a Scripture, refer to the "My Identity In Christ" exercise on page 107.) Lastly, combine what you like about yourself, how it makes you feel, and the Scripture reinforcement into a positive phrase.

| WHAT I LIKE ABOUT MYSELF: | IT MAKES ME FEEL… | SCRIPTURE THAT REINFORCES THIS: | POSITIVE SELF-TALK PHRASE: |
|---|---|---|---|
| *I like that I help people with their house projects.* | *It makes me feel kind, productive, and needed.* | *Psalm 145:17 - modeling the kindness of God* | *I show kindness when I'm helpful in practically meeting the needs of others.* |
| | | | |

[33] *What About Bob?*, directed by Frank Oz (Burbank: Touchstone Pictures, 1991), film.

| WHAT I LIKE ABOUT MYSELF: | IT MAKES ME FEEL… | SCRIPTURE THAT REINFORCES THIS: | POSITIVE SELF-TALK PHRASE: |
|---|---|---|---|
| | | | |
| | | | |
| | | | |
| | | | |

**Give yourself time this week to practice saying this phrase out loud.** This is a great way to engage another part of your brain, your auditory system, which will help to make positive self-talk part of your thought process.

Developing positive self-talk can help to silence our inner critic and change the way we think about ourselves, so that we begin to see ourselves the way God sees us. One of the main goals of the Hero's Journey is to discover who we are in Christ and become the man (husband, father, leader) God created us to be.

# FASTER Scale

> Circle the behaviors on the FASTER Scale that you identify with in each section.
> Identify the most powerful behavior in each section and write it next to the corresponding heading.
> Answer the following three questions based on your most powerful or frequent behavior.

01. How does it affect me? How do I feel in the moment?
02. How does it affect the important people in my life?
03. Why do I do this? What is the benefit for me?

## RESTORATION ____________________

*(Accepting life on God's terms, with trust, grace, mercy, vulnerability and gratitude.)* No current secrets; working to resolve problems; identifying fears and feelings; keeping commitments to meetings, prayer, family, church, people, goals, and self; being open and honest, making eye contact; increasing in relationships with God and others; true accountability.

01. ____________________
02. ____________________
03. ____________________

## FORGETTING PRIORITIES ____________________

*(Start believing the present circumstances and moving away from trusting God. Denial; flight; a change in what's important; how you spend your time, energy, and thoughts.)* Secrets; less time/energy for God, meetings, church; avoiding support and accountability people; superficial conversations; sarcasm; isolating; changes in goals; obsessed with relationships; breaking promises and commitments; neglecting family; preoccupation with material things, TV, computers, entertainment; procrastination; lying; overconfidence; bored; hiding money; image management; seeking to control situations and other people.

01. ____________________
____________________
02. ____________________
____________________
03. ____________________
____________________

## ANXIETY

*(Consumed by negative thoughts and undefined fear; getting energy from emotions.)* Worry, using profanity, being fearful; being resentful; replaying old, negative thoughts; perfectionism; judging other's motives; making goals and lists that you can't complete; mind reading; fantasy, codependent, rescuing; sleep problems, trouble concentrating, seeking/creating drama; gossip; using over-the-counter medication for pain, sleep or weight control; flirting.

01. ______________________

02. ______________________

03. ______________________

## SPEEDING UP

*(Trying to outrun the anxiety which is usually the first sign of depression.)* Super busy and always in a hurry (finding good reason to justify the work); workaholic; can't relax; avoiding slowing down; feeling driven; can't turn off thoughts; skipping meals; binge eating (usually at night); overspending; can't identify own feelings/needs; repetitive negative thoughts; irritable; dramatic mood swings; too much caffeine; over exercising; nervousness; difficulty being alone and/or with people; difficulty listening to others; making excuses for having to "do it all."

01. ______________________

02. ______________________

03. ______________________

## TICKED OFF

*(Getting adrenaline high on anger and aggression.)* Procrastination causing crisis in money, work, and relationships; increased sarcasm; black and white (all or nothing) thinking; feeling alone; nobody understands; overreacting, road rage; constant resentments; pushing others away; increasing isolation; blaming; arguing; irrational thinking; can't take criticism; defensive; people avoiding you; needing to be right; digestive problems; headaches; obsessive (stuck) thoughts; can't forgive; feeling superior; using intimidation.

01. ______________________________________________

______________________________________________

02. ______________________________________________

______________________________________________

03. ______________________________________________

______________________________________________

## EXHAUSTED ______________________________________________

*(Loss of physical and emotional energy; coming off the adrenaline high, and the onset of depression.)* Depressed; panicked; confused; hopelessness; sleeping too much or too little; can't cope; overwhelmed; crying for "no reason"; can't think; forgetful; pessimistic; helpless; tired; numb; wanting to run; constant cravings for old coping behaviors; thinking of using sex, drugs, or alcohol; seeking old unhealthy people and places; really isolating; people angry with you; self abuse; suicidal thoughts; spontaneous crying; no goals; survival mode; not returning phone calls; missing work; irritability; no appetite.

01. ______________________________________________

______________________________________________

02. ______________________________________________

______________________________________________

03. ______________________________________________

______________________________________________

## RELAPSE ______________________________________________

*(Returning to the place you swore you would never go again. Coping with life on your terms. You sitting in the driver's seat instead of God.)* Giving up and giving in; out of control; lost in your addiction; lying to yourself and others; feeling you just can't manage without your coping behaviors, at least for now. The result is the reinforcement of shame, guilt and condemnation; and feelings of abandonment and being alone.

01. ______________________________________________

______________________________________________

02. ______________________________________________

______________________________________________

03. ______________________________________________

______________________________________________

# Commitment To Change

Complete the Commitment to Change prior to your next group meeting.

Keep in mind, your Commitment to Change is often directly connected to the lowest level reached on the FASTER Scale. Healing happens best when we are fully aware of the challenges we face and take proactive steps to create change.

## LET'S PLAN FOR NEXT WEEK

### Commitment to change: what area do you need to change or what challenge are you facing this week?

- Double bind: what will it cost you if you change? If you don't change?
- How does this potential for change make you feel?
- What is your plan to maintain restoration regarding these changes?

### Who will you share your commitment with this week?

### What are the details of your accountability? What questions should they ask you?

**BE PREPARED TO SHARE YOUR ANSWERS IN THIS CHAPTER WITH THE GUYS IN YOUR GROUP.**

CHAPTER 18

# DEFINING MY NEW NORMAL

## Group Check-In

Complete the Group Check-In 24 hours before group.

### HOW DID YOU DO LAST WEEK?

01. How did you do on your Commitment to Change? ______

02. Did you lie directly or indirectly to anyone? ______

03. What did you do to improve significant relationships with your wife, family, or friends? ______

### WHERE ARE YOU RIGHT NOW?

04. What is the lowest level you identify with on the FASTER Scale? ______

# Building Resiliency

Lifelong healing happens when we are proactive, applying everything we've learned to the way we live out each day of our lives. When life is great, this is an easy task because of the way we've trained ourselves to focus on the things we need to do and say to stay healthy. But when life feels challenging and we're bombarded by chaotic and negative thoughts, it can be much more difficult to focus on the things we need to do and say to stay healthy. In situations like this, we are more likely to feel overwhelmed and out of control, which often leads to relapse.

So what do we do? How do we maintain health and walk through a difficult situation at the same time? The answer: practice, practice, and more practice.

The more we train ourselves—train our brain—to function in a healthy way, the more resilient we become and better equipped to quickly bounce back when life is challenging.

Many of us have the capacity to think and behave rationally when faced with various situations. But when caught up in a difficult situation or difficult season of life, our negative or irrational thoughts and feelings get in the way of us doing what we know will help us. This is why we need to develop a mindset for health that includes intentionally processing situations and practicing a response. Much like an athlete mentally rehearses before a big game and focuses on seeing themselves perform well, they will be more successful during the game.

Practicing helps us to restructure and change our irrational or unhealthy thought processes and behavioral patterns. The more we practice and train ourselves, the more resilient we become over time.

The ABCDE Model is a useful tool for processing difficult situations and practicing a healthy response.[34] Each letter represents a step (or steps) in this process. Here's how it works.

- **A:** the **activating event** or situation creating problems or issues in your life. This could include a traumatic event, a relationship, a situation out of your control but impacting you, and many other possibilities.
- **B:** your **beliefs** and thoughts about the activating event (A).
- **C:** the **consequences** of your beliefs (B) about the activating event (A). This often results in emotional, behavioral, and thought processes, both negative (disruptive) and positive (goal oriented).
- **D:** when you question or **dispute** your beliefs. This may include identifying your irrational or unreasonable beliefs, as well as identifying constructive and rational thoughts to help override any distorted thought patterns.

---

[34] Stephanie Wright, "All About Rational Emotive Behavior Therapy (REBT)," PsychCentral, April 15,2022, https://psychcentral.com/lib/rational-emotive-behavior-therapy.

- **E:** where you develop **effective behaviors**. This comes from evaluating what you've learned and making proactive changes to help you best manage similar situations in the future.

## ABCDE Model[35]

In the following table,

- write a brief description of the activating event or situation (A).
- identify your beliefs about the event or situation, both your irrational beliefs and your rational beliefs (B). Identifying an alternative rational belief will help you create more goal oriented consequences.
- list the consequences of your beliefs (C): it may be easier to first identify your emotional distress, dysfunctional behaviors, and distorted thinking before identifying your emotional, behavioral, and thinking goals. Identifying your beliefs and consequences are interchangeable; B then C or C then B.
- argue with yourself. When disputing your beliefs, you're persuading yourself that your irrational beliefs are irrational and convincing yourself that your rational beliefs are rational. This will also help you create and achieve your emotional, behavioral, and thinking goals for future situations.
- evaluate your response to this situation. Given everything you know now, if there's a better way to handle a similar activating event or situation (A) in the future, what would it look like?

*Example:*

| **A - Activating event or situation:** |
| --- |
| A position opened up at the company where I've worked for 10 years. I met all the preferred qualifications for the job, so I applied for it. If I got this job, it would mean a promotion and a pay increase. I went through the interview process, which seemed to go well. Or so I thought. I didn't get the job. They hired someone from outside the company who had far less experience than me. |

[35] Keith S. Dobson, *Handbook of Cognitive Behavioral Therapies*, 3rd ed. (New York: The Guilford Press, 2010), 253.

| **B - Belief about A (irrational belief):** I will never be good enough. My mom was right, I'm always going to be a loser just like my dad. I'll never be successful and have the good things in life. | **B - Belief about A (rational belief):** I'm smart and a good worker. I'm successful in a lot of areas. This is not about my abilities but about trusting God's plan for my life. |
|---|---|
| **C - Consequence to B (emotional/distress):** angry, confused, disappointed, aggressive, desperate, hopeless. | **C - Consequence to B (emotion/goal):** grateful, energized, creative, hopeful. |
| **C - Consequence to B (behavior/dysfunction):** I was so angry and disappointed when I got home, I yelled at my kids, ignored my wife, and isolated myself by playing video games in my room. | **C - Consequence to B (behavior/goal):** I went home and talked with my wife. We decided to make a special family dinner and celebrate all the wonderful things we have to be thankful for in our life. |
| **C - Consequence to B (thinking/distorted):** Why can't I get a break? That guy is no better than me. This is how my life will always be. I'm a loser and alone. I always have been and always will be. | **C - Consequence to B (thinking/goal):** I'm very capable and a hard worker. I am successful in many areas of my life. I will apply for opportunities when they come up and follow God's leading. |

**D - Disputing:**

You are good enough. You are smart and graduated top in your class. Your family loves you; you're a great husband and father! You have a strong community of friends who love and support you. You're a hard worker. You're not a loser. God has bigger plans for you than this job. Be patient and trust Him. He'll show you the way.

**E - Effective behavior:**

If I apply for a job and don't get it, it's not personally against me. Even if I feel disappointed, I will focus on being proactive with my thoughts, feelings, and behaviors. I will not take out my disappointments on those around me but will engage in community with those who love and support me.

Now it's your turn. Use the above instructions to fill in the following table. Take your time. Be intentional about describing the details within each step and determining what proactive behaviors would be helpful in building resiliency.

| **A - Activating event or situation:** | |
|---|---|
| **B - Belief about A (irrational belief):** | **B - Belief about A (rational belief):** |
| **C - Consequence to B (emotional/distress):** | **C - Consequence to B (emotion/goal):** |
| **C - Consequence to B (behavior/dysfunction):** | **C - Consequence to B (behavior/goal):** |

| C - Consequence to B (thinking/distorted): | C - Consequence to B (thinking/goal): |
| --- | --- |
| D - Disputing: | |
| E - Effective behavior: | |

Building resiliency is an important part of our healing journey. It's a way of training ourselves and our brain to choose a better way, a healthy way of navigating the challenging aspects of life. It equips us to handle future situations in a way that benefits us and those around us.

# FASTER Scale

Circle the behaviors on the FASTER Scale that you identify with in each section.
Identify the most powerful behavior in each section and write it next to the corresponding heading.
Answer the following three questions based on your most powerful or frequent behavior.

01. How does it affect me? How do I feel in the moment?
02. How does it affect the important people in my life?
03. Why do I do this? What is the benefit for me?

## RESTORATION ______________________________

*(Accepting life on God's terms, with trust, grace, mercy, vulnerability and gratitude.)* No current secrets; working to resolve problems; identifying fears and feelings; keeping commitments to meetings, prayer, family, church, people, goals, and self; being open and honest, making eye contact; increasing in relationships with God and others; true accountability.

01. ______________________________
02. ______________________________
03. ______________________________

## FORGETTING PRIORITIES ______________________________

*(Start believing the present circumstances and moving away from trusting God. Denial; flight; a change in what's important; how you spend your time, energy, and thoughts.)* Secrets; less time/energy for God, meetings, church; avoiding support and accountability people; superficial conversations; sarcasm; isolating; changes in goals; obsessed with relationships; breaking promises and commitments; neglecting family; preoccupation with material things, TV, computers, entertainment; procrastination; lying; overconfidence; bored; hiding money; image management; seeking to control situations and other people.

01. ______________________________
______________________________
02. ______________________________
______________________________
03. ______________________________
______________________________

## ANXIETY

*(Consumed by negative thoughts and undefined fear; getting energy from emotions.)* Worry, using profanity, being fearful; being resentful; replaying old, negative thoughts; perfectionism; judging other's motives; making goals and lists that you can't complete; mind reading; fantasy, codependent, rescuing; sleep problems, trouble concentrating, seeking/creating drama; gossip; using over-the-counter medication for pain, sleep or weight control; flirting.

01. ______________________________

02. ______________________________

03. ______________________________

## SPEEDING UP

*(Trying to outrun the anxiety which is usually the first sign of depression.)* Super busy and always in a hurry (finding good reason to justify the work); workaholic; can't relax; avoiding slowing down; feeling driven; can't turn off thoughts; skipping meals; binge eating (usually at night); overspending; can't identify own feelings/needs; repetitive negative thoughts; irritable; dramatic mood swings; too much caffeine; over exercising; nervousness; difficulty being alone and/or with people; difficulty listening to others; making excuses for having to "do it all."

01. ______________________________

02. ______________________________

03. ______________________________

## TICKED OFF

*(Getting adrenaline high on anger and aggression.)* Procrastination causing crisis in money, work, and relationships; increased sarcasm; black and white (all or nothing) thinking; feeling alone; nobody understands; overreacting, road rage; constant resentments; pushing others away; increasing isolation; blaming; arguing; irrational thinking; can't take criticism; defensive; people avoiding you; needing to be right; digestive problems; headaches; obsessive (stuck) thoughts; can't forgive; feeling superior; using intimidation.

01.

02.

03.

## EXHAUSTED

*(Loss of physical and emotional energy; coming off the adrenaline high, and the onset of depression.)* Depressed; panicked; confused; hopelessness; sleeping too much or too little; can't cope; overwhelmed; crying for "no reason"; can't think; forgetful; pessimistic; helpless; tired; numb; wanting to run; constant cravings for old coping behaviors; thinking of using sex, drugs, or alcohol; seeking old unhealthy people and places; really isolating; people angry with you; self abuse; suicidal thoughts; spontaneous crying; no goals; survival mode; not returning phone calls; missing work; irritability; no appetite.

01.

02.

03.

## RELAPSE

*(Returning to the place you swore you would never go again. Coping with life on your terms. You sitting in the driver's seat instead of God.)* Giving up and giving in; out of control; lost in your addiction; lying to yourself and others; feeling you just can't manage without your coping behaviors, at least for now. The result is the reinforcement of shame, guilt and condemnation; and feelings of abandonment and being alone.

01.

02.

03.

# Commitment To Change

Complete the Commitment to Change prior to your next group meeting.

Keep in mind, your Commitment to Change is often directly connected to the lowest level reached on the FASTER Scale. Healing happens best when we are fully aware of the challenges we face and take proactive steps to create change.

## LET'S PLAN FOR NEXT WEEK

### Commitment to change: what area do you need to change or what challenge are you facing this week?

- Double bind: what will it cost you if you change? If you don't change?
- How does this potential for change make you feel?
- What is your plan to maintain restoration regarding these changes?

### Who will you share your commitment with this week?

### What are the details of your accountability? What questions should they ask you?

BE PREPARED TO SHARE YOUR ANSWERS IN THIS CHAPTER WITH THE GUYS IN YOUR GROUP.

CHAPTER 19

# STUMBLING INTO GREATNESS

## Group Check-In

Complete the Group Check-In 24 hours before group.

### HOW DID YOU DO LAST WEEK?

01. How did you do on your Commitment to Change? ______

02. Did you lie directly or indirectly to anyone? ______

03. What did you do to improve significant relationships with your wife, family, or friends? ______

### WHERE ARE YOU RIGHT NOW?

04. What is the lowest level you identify with on the FASTER Scale? ______

# The Strength of Relationship

When you were first married, you probably loved everything about your wife. Yet over time, the things you loved about her became commonplace and now you take for granted all the amazing things she does for you.

When this happens, it can be helpful to think about all the things you love about your wife and the shared experiences where this has strengthened your relationship.

**On the following list, circle at least five qualities you love most about your wife.[36] If you are not yet married, what qualities are you looking for in a spouse? Circle at least five qualities you would like in a spouse.** Referring to your A-Z list in Chapter 16 might be a helpful starting place.

**She is...**

- Adventurous
- Ambitious
- Artistic
- Assertive
- Athletic
- Brave
- Conscientious
- Confident
- Cooperative
- Creative
- Curious
- Disciplined
- Empathic
- Energetic
- Enthusiastic
- Fair
- Flexible
- Forgiving
- Grateful
- Honest
- Humorous
- Independent
- Intelligent
- Kind
- Leader
- Logical
- Loving
- Modest
- Nurturing
- Open Minded
- Optimistic
- Passionate
- Patient
- Persistent
- Self-Controlled
- Spontaneous
- Stable
- Spiritual
- Thoughtful
- Wise

---

36 Couple's Strengths Exploration, TherapistAid.com, 2020. https://www.therapistaid.com/worksheets/couples-strengths-exploration.

In the following space, identify the top three qualities you circled; for each one, share a memory where your wife demonstrated this quality toward you and how it strengthened your relationship. If you're not married, share why you hope your future wife has this quality.

## STRENGTH #1:

***I remember...*** Or ***I hope...***

## STRENGTH #2:

***I remember...*** Or ***I hope...***

## STRENGTH #3:

***I remember...*** Or ***I hope...***

Your wife is a precious gift from God. Even during difficult times, God gave you the perfect wife for you. Remember the wonderful things she does for you and how she brings strength to your relationship.

# FASTER Scale

Circle the behaviors on the FASTER Scale that you identify with in each section.
Identify the most powerful behavior in each section and write it next to the corresponding heading.
Answer the following three questions based on your most powerful or frequent behavior.

01. How does it affect me? How do I feel in the moment?
02. How does it affect the important people in my life?
03. Why do I do this? What is the benefit for me?

## RESTORATION ______

*(Accepting life on God's terms, with trust, grace, mercy, vulnerability and gratitude.)* No current secrets; working to resolve problems; identifying fears and feelings; keeping commitments to meetings, prayer, family, church, people, goals, and self; being open and honest, making eye contact; increasing in relationships with God and others; true accountability.

01. ______
02. ______
03. ______

## FORGETTING PRIORITIES ______

*(Start believing the present circumstances and moving away from trusting God. Denial; flight; a change in what's important; how you spend your time, energy, and thoughts.)* Secrets; less time/energy for God, meetings, church; avoiding support and accountability people; superficial conversations; sarcasm; isolating; changes in goals; obsessed with relationships; breaking promises and commitments; neglecting family; preoccupation with material things, TV, computers, entertainment; procrastination; lying; overconfidence; bored; hiding money; image management; seeking to control situations and other people.

01. ______
______
02. ______
______
03. ______
______

## ANXIETY

*(Consumed by negative thoughts and undefined fear; getting energy from emotions.)* Worry, using profanity, being fearful; being resentful; replaying old, negative thoughts; perfectionism; judging other's motives; making goals and lists that you can't complete; mind reading; fantasy, codependent, rescuing; sleep problems, trouble concentrating, seeking/creating drama; gossip; using over-the-counter medication for pain, sleep or weight control; flirting.

01. ____________________

02. ____________________

03. ____________________

## SPEEDING UP

*(Trying to outrun the anxiety which is usually the first sign of depression.)* Super busy and always in a hurry (finding good reason to justify the work); workaholic; can't relax; avoiding slowing down; feeling driven; can't turn off thoughts; skipping meals; binge eating (usually at night); overspending; can't identify own feelings/needs; repetitive negative thoughts; irritable; dramatic mood swings; too much caffeine; over exercising; nervousness; difficulty being alone and/or with people; difficulty listening to others; making excuses for having to "do it all."

01. ____________________

02. ____________________

03. ____________________

## TICKED OFF

*(Getting adrenaline high on anger and aggression.)* Procrastination causing crisis in money, work, and relationships; increased sarcasm; black and white (all or nothing) thinking; feeling alone; nobody understands; overreacting, road rage; constant resentments; pushing others away; increasing isolation; blaming; arguing; irrational thinking; can't take criticism; defensive; people avoiding you; needing to be right; digestive problems; headaches; obsessive (stuck) thoughts; can't forgive; feeling superior; using intimidation.

01.

02.

03.

## EXHAUSTED

*(Loss of physical and emotional energy; coming off the adrenaline high, and the onset of depression.)* Depressed; panicked; confused; hopelessness; sleeping too much or too little; can't cope; overwhelmed; crying for "no reason"; can't think; forgetful; pessimistic; helpless; tired; numb; wanting to run; constant cravings for old coping behaviors; thinking of using sex, drugs, or alcohol; seeking old unhealthy people and places; really isolating; people angry with you; self abuse; suicidal thoughts; spontaneous crying; no goals; survival mode; not returning phone calls; missing work; irritability; no appetite.

01.

02.

03.

## RELAPSE

*(Returning to the place you swore you would never go again. Coping with life on your terms. You sitting in the driver's seat instead of God.)* Giving up and giving in; out of control; lost in your addiction; lying to yourself and others; feeling you just can't manage without your coping behaviors, at least for now. The result is the reinforcement of shame, guilt and condemnation; and feelings of abandonment and being alone.

01.

02.

03.

# Commitment To Change

Complete the Commitment to Change prior to your next group meeting.

Keep in mind, your Commitment to Change is often directly connected to the lowest level reached on the FASTER Scale. Healing happens best when we are fully aware of the challenges we face and take proactive steps to create change.

## LET'S PLAN FOR NEXT WEEK

### Commitment to change: what area do you need to change or what challenge are you facing this week?

- Double bind: what will it cost you if you change? If you don't change?
- How does this potential for change make you feel?
- What is your plan to maintain restoration regarding these changes?

### Who will you share your commitment with this week?

### What are the details of your accountability? What questions should they ask you?

BE PREPARED TO SHARE YOUR ANSWERS IN THIS CHAPTER WITH THE GUYS IN YOUR GROUP.

STAGE VIII

# WRAP UP

## What do you think?

> This has been an incredible journey! What was the most significant change you've experienced? What area challenged you most? What tool or practice will you incorporate into your daily life? How did this experience change your relationships with the people closest to you (wife, kids, family, friends)?

# Progress, not Perfection

This journey doesn't stop here. Throughout our lifetime we will continue to change and grow. This is the nature of progress. What continue to be the most impactful small steps you're taking toward healing? All of these small steps are helping you become a Compassionate Warrior and leading you to the life God has for you.

| ISSUE | PERFECTION | WHERE I STARTED | PROGRESS |
|---|---|---|---|
| | | | |

What can you do this week to make progress toward your goal?

| ISSUE | PERFECTION | WHERE I STARTED | PROGRESS |
|---|---|---|---|
| | | | |

What can you do this week to make progress toward your goal?

| ISSUE | PERFECTION | WHERE I STARTED | PROGRESS |
|---|---|---|---|
| | | | |

What can you do this week to make progress toward your goal?

## Thoughts & Feelings Awareness Log

Learning to identify your thoughts and feelings is equipping you to be more emotionally aware; not only aware of your own feelings, but also aware of the feelings of others. This is what becoming a Compassionate Warrior is all about.

| I FELT... | ...BECAUSE I THOUGHT... |
|---|---|
| | |
| | |
| | |

The journaling and tools in this wrap up are for you, so you can evaluate what you're learning and keep track of the progress you're making. You don't have to share any of this with the guys in your group, but can if you want to.

# CONCLUSION
# CLOSING COMMENTS

## Group Check-In

Complete the Group Check-In 24 hours before group.

### HOW DID YOU DO LAST WEEK?

01. How did you do on your Commitment to Change? ______________________

02. Did you lie directly or indirectly to anyone? ______________________

03. What did you do to improve significant relationships with your wife, family, or friends? ______________________

### WHERE ARE YOU RIGHT NOW?

04. What is the lowest level you identify with on the FASTER Scale? ______________________

# FASTER Scale

Circle the behaviors on the FASTER Scale that you identify with in each section.
Identify the most powerful behavior in each section and write it next to the corresponding heading.
Answer the following three questions based on your most powerful or frequent behavior.

01. How does it affect me? How do I feel in the moment?
02. How does it affect the important people in my life?
03. Why do I do this? What is the benefit for me?

## RESTORATION ______________________________

*(Accepting life on God's terms, with trust, grace, mercy, vulnerability and gratitude.)* No current secrets; working to resolve problems; identifying fears and feelings; keeping commitments to meetings, prayer, family, church, people, goals, and self; being open and honest, making eye contact; increasing in relationships with God and others; true accountability.

01. ______________________________
02. ______________________________
03. ______________________________

## FORGETTING PRIORITIES ______________________________

*(Start believing the present circumstances and moving away from trusting God. Denial; flight; a change in what's important; how you spend your time, energy, and thoughts.)* Secrets; less time/energy for God, meetings, church; avoiding support and accountability people; superficial conversations; sarcasm; isolating; changes in goals; obsessed with relationships; breaking promises and commitments; neglecting family; preoccupation with material things, TV, computers, entertainment; procrastination; lying; overconfidence; bored; hiding money; image management; seeking to control situations and other people.

01. ______________________________
______________________________
02. ______________________________
______________________________
03. ______________________________
______________________________

## ANXIETY

*(Consumed by negative thoughts and undefined fear; getting energy from emotions.)* Worry, using profanity, being fearful; being resentful; replaying old, negative thoughts; perfectionism; judging other's motives; making goals and lists that you can't complete; mind reading; fantasy, codependent, rescuing; sleep problems, trouble concentrating, seeking/creating drama; gossip; using over-the-counter medication for pain, sleep or weight control; flirting.

01. ______________________________

02. ______________________________

03. ______________________________

## SPEEDING UP

*(Trying to outrun the anxiety which is usually the first sign of depression.)* Super busy and always in a hurry (finding good reason to justify the work); workaholic; can't relax; avoiding slowing down; feeling driven; can't turn off thoughts; skipping meals; binge eating (usually at night); overspending; can't identify own feelings/needs; repetitive negative thoughts; irritable; dramatic mood swings; too much caffeine; over exercising; nervousness; difficulty being alone and/or with people; difficulty listening to others; making excuses for having to "do it all."

01. ______________________________

02. ______________________________

03. ______________________________

## TICKED OFF

*(Getting adrenaline high on anger and aggression.)* Procrastination causing crisis in money, work, and relationships; increased sarcasm; black and white (all or nothing) thinking; feeling alone; nobody understands; overreacting, road rage; constant resentments; pushing others away; increasing isolation; blaming; arguing; irrational thinking; can't take criticism; defensive; people avoiding you; needing to be right; digestive problems; headaches; obsessive (stuck) thoughts; can't forgive; feeling superior; using intimidation.

01. ____________________

____________________

02. ____________________

____________________

03. ____________________

____________________

## EXHAUSTED ____________________

*(Loss of physical and emotional energy; coming off the adrenaline high, and the onset of depression.)* Depressed; panicked; confused; hopelessness; sleeping too much or too little; can't cope; overwhelmed; crying for "no reason"; can't think; forgetful; pessimistic; helpless; tired; numb; wanting to run; constant cravings for old coping behaviors; thinking of using sex, drugs, or alcohol; seeking old unhealthy people and places; really isolating; people angry with you; self abuse; suicidal thoughts; spontaneous crying; no goals; survival mode; not returning phone calls; missing work; irritability; no appetite.

01. ____________________

____________________

02. ____________________

____________________

03. ____________________

____________________

## RELAPSE ____________________

*(Returning to the place you swore you would never go again. Coping with life on your terms. You sitting in the driver's seat instead of God.)* Giving up and giving in; out of control; lost in your addiction; lying to yourself and others; feeling you just can't manage without your coping behaviors, at least for now. The result is the reinforcement of shame, guilt and condemnation; and feelings of abandonment and being alone.

01. ____________________

____________________

02. ____________________

____________________

03. ____________________

____________________

# Commitment To Change

Complete the Commitment to Change prior to your next group meeting.

Keep in mind, your Commitment to Change is often directly connected to the lowest level reached on the FASTER Scale. Healing happens best when we are fully aware of the challenges we face and take proactive steps to create change.

## LET'S PLAN FOR NEXT WEEK

Commitment to change: what area do you need to change or what challenge are you facing this week?

- Double bind: what will it cost you if you change? If you don't change?
- How does this potential for change make you feel?
- What is your plan to maintain restoration regarding these changes?

Who will you share your commitment with this week?

What are the details of your accountability? What questions should they ask you?

BE PREPARED TO SHARE YOUR ANSWERS IN THIS CHAPTER WITH THE GUYS IN YOUR GROUP.

# APPENDIX
# WEEK ______

All of the tools you need for each week are included within each chapter. However, you may encounter weeks where you run out of time and need to extend the week's work over two weeks. We've added additional tools in case this happens within your group experience.

## Group Check-In

Complete the Group Check-In 24 hours before group.

### HOW DID YOU DO LAST WEEK?

01. How did you do on your Commitment to Change? ______

02. Did you lie directly or indirectly to anyone? ______

03. What did you do to improve significant relationships with your wife, family, or friends? ______

### WHERE ARE YOU RIGHT NOW?

04. What is the lowest level you identify with on the FASTER Scale? ______

# FASTER Scale

Circle the behaviors on the FASTER Scale that you identify with in each section.
Identify the most powerful behavior in each section and write it next to the corresponding heading.
Answer the following three questions based on your most powerful or frequent behavior.

01. How does it affect me? How do I feel in the moment?
02. How does it affect the important people in my life?
03. Why do I do this? What is the benefit for me?

## RESTORATION ______________________________

*(Accepting life on God's terms, with trust, grace, mercy, vulnerability and gratitude.)* No current secrets; working to resolve problems; identifying fears and feelings; keeping commitments to meetings, prayer, family, church, people, goals, and self; being open and honest, making eye contact; increasing in relationships with God and others; true accountability.

01. ______________________________
02. ______________________________
03. ______________________________

## FORGETTING PRIORITIES ______________________________

*(Start believing the present circumstances and moving away from trusting God. Denial; flight; a change in what's important; how you spend your time, energy, and thoughts.)* Secrets; less time/energy for God, meetings, church; avoiding support and accountability people; superficial conversations; sarcasm; isolating; changes in goals; obsessed with relationships; breaking promises and commitments; neglecting family; preoccupation with material things, TV, computers, entertainment; procrastination; lying; overconfidence; bored; hiding money; image management; seeking to control situations and other people.

01. ______________________________
______________________________
02. ______________________________
______________________________
03. ______________________________
______________________________

## ANXIETY

*(Consumed by negative thoughts and undefined fear; getting energy from emotions.)* Worry, using profanity, being fearful; being resentful; replaying old, negative thoughts; perfectionism; judging other's motives; making goals and lists that you can't complete; mind reading; fantasy, codependent, rescuing; sleep problems, trouble concentrating, seeking/creating drama; gossip; using over-the-counter medication for pain, sleep or weight control; flirting.

01. ______

02. ______

03. ______

## SPEEDING UP

*(Trying to outrun the anxiety which is usually the first sign of depression.)* Super busy and always in a hurry (finding good reason to justify the work); workaholic; can't relax; avoiding slowing down; feeling driven; can't turn off thoughts; skipping meals; binge eating (usually at night); overspending; can't identify own feelings/needs; repetitive negative thoughts; irritable; dramatic mood swings; too much caffeine; over exercising; nervousness; difficulty being alone and/or with people; difficulty listening to others; making excuses for having to "do it all."

01. ______

02. ______

03. ______

## TICKED OFF

*(Getting adrenaline high on anger and aggression.)* Procrastination causing crisis in money, work, and relationships; increased sarcasm; black and white (all or nothing) thinking; feeling alone; nobody understands; overreacting, road rage; constant resentments; pushing others away; increasing isolation; blaming; arguing; irrational thinking; can't take criticism; defensive; people avoiding you; needing to be right; digestive problems; headaches; obsessive (stuck) thoughts; can't forgive; feeling superior; using intimidation.

01. ______________________________

______________________________

02. ______________________________

______________________________

03. ______________________________

______________________________

## EXHAUSTED ______________________________

*(Loss of physical and emotional energy; coming off the adrenaline high, and the onset of depression.)* Depressed; panicked; confused; hopelessness; sleeping too much or too little; can't cope; overwhelmed; crying for "no reason"; can't think; forgetful; pessimistic; helpless; tired; numb; wanting to run; constant cravings for old coping behaviors; thinking of using sex, drugs, or alcohol; seeking old unhealthy people and places; really isolating; people angry with you; self abuse; suicidal thoughts; spontaneous crying; no goals; survival mode; not returning phone calls; missing work; irritability; no appetite.

01. ______________________________

______________________________

02. ______________________________

______________________________

03. ______________________________

______________________________

## RELAPSE ______________________________

*(Returning to the place you swore you would never go again. Coping with life on your terms. You sitting in the driver's seat instead of God.)* Giving up and giving in; out of control; lost in your addiction; lying to yourself and others; feeling you just can't manage without your coping behaviors, at least for now. The result is the reinforcement of shame, guilt and condemnation; and feelings of abandonment and being alone.

01. ______________________________

______________________________

02. ______________________________

______________________________

03. ______________________________

______________________________

# Commitment To Change

Complete the Commitment to Change prior to your next group meeting.

Keep in mind, your Commitment to Change is often directly connected to the lowest level reached on the FASTER Scale. Healing happens best when we are fully aware of the challenges we face and take proactive steps to create change.

## LET'S PLAN FOR NEXT WEEK

### Commitment to change: what area do you need to change or what challenge are you facing this week?

- Double bind: what will it cost you if you change? If you don't change?
- How does this potential for change make you feel?
- What is your plan to maintain restoration regarding these changes?

### Who will you share your commitment with this week?

### What are the details of your accountability? What questions should they ask you?

BE PREPARED TO SHARE YOUR ANSWERS IN THIS CHAPTER WITH THE GUYS IN YOUR GROUP.

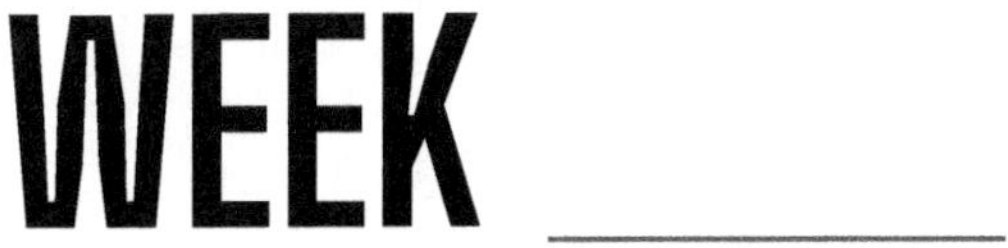

## Group Check-In

Complete the Group Check-In 24 hours before group.

### HOW DID YOU DO LAST WEEK?

01. How did you do on your Commitment to Change?

02. Did you lie directly or indirectly to anyone?

03. What did you do to improve significant relationships with your wife, family, or friends?

### WHERE ARE YOU RIGHT NOW?

04. What is the lowest level you identify with on the FASTER Scale?

# FASTER Scale

Circle the behaviors on the FASTER Scale that you identify with in each section.
Identify the most powerful behavior in each section and write it next to the corresponding heading.
Answer the following three questions based on your most powerful or frequent behavior.

01. How does it affect me? How do I feel in the moment?
02. How does it affect the important people in my life?
03. Why do I do this? What is the benefit for me?

## RESTORATION ____________________

*(Accepting life on God's terms, with trust, grace, mercy, vulnerability and gratitude.)* No current secrets; working to resolve problems; identifying fears and feelings; keeping commitments to meetings, prayer, family, church, people, goals, and self; being open and honest, making eye contact; increasing in relationships with God and others; true accountability.

01. ____________________
02. ____________________
03. ____________________

## FORGETTING PRIORITIES ____________________

*(Start believing the present circumstances and moving away from trusting God. Denial; flight; a change in what's important; how you spend your time, energy, and thoughts.)* Secrets; less time/energy for God, meetings, church; avoiding support and accountability people; superficial conversations; sarcasm; isolating; changes in goals; obsessed with relationships; breaking promises and commitments; neglecting family; preoccupation with material things, TV, computers, entertainment; procrastination; lying; overconfidence; bored; hiding money; image management; seeking to control situations and other people.

01. ____________________
____________________
02. ____________________
____________________
03. ____________________
____________________

## ANXIETY

*(Consumed by negative thoughts and undefined fear; getting energy from emotions.)* Worry, using profanity, being fearful; being resentful; replaying old, negative thoughts; perfectionism; judging other's motives; making goals and lists that you can't complete; mind reading; fantasy, codependent, rescuing; sleep problems, trouble concentrating, seeking/creating drama; gossip; using over-the-counter medication for pain, sleep or weight control; flirting.

01. ______

02. ______

03. ______

## SPEEDING UP

*(Trying to outrun the anxiety which is usually the first sign of depression.)* Super busy and always in a hurry (finding good reason to justify the work); workaholic; can't relax; avoiding slowing down; feeling driven; can't turn off thoughts; skipping meals; binge eating (usually at night); overspending; can't identify own feelings/needs; repetitive negative thoughts; irritable; dramatic mood swings; too much caffeine; over exercising; nervousness; difficulty being alone and/or with people; difficulty listening to others; making excuses for having to "do it all."

01. ______

02. ______

03. ______

## TICKED OFF

*(Getting adrenaline high on anger and aggression.)* Procrastination causing crisis in money, work, and relationships; increased sarcasm; black and white (all or nothing) thinking; feeling alone; nobody understands; overreacting, road rage; constant resentments; pushing others away; increasing isolation; blaming; arguing; irrational thinking; can't take criticism; defensive; people avoiding you; needing to be right; digestive problems; headaches; obsessive (stuck) thoughts; can't forgive; feeling superior; using intimidation.

01. ______________________________

______________________________

02. ______________________________

______________________________

03. ______________________________

______________________________

## EXHAUSTED ______________________________

*(Loss of physical and emotional energy; coming off the adrenaline high, and the onset of depression.)* Depressed; panicked; confused; hopelessness; sleeping too much or too little; can't cope; overwhelmed; crying for "no reason"; can't think; forgetful; pessimistic; helpless; tired; numb; wanting to run; constant cravings for old coping behaviors; thinking of using sex, drugs, or alcohol; seeking old unhealthy people and places; really isolating; people angry with you; self abuse; suicidal thoughts; spontaneous crying; no goals; survival mode; not returning phone calls; missing work; irritability; no appetite.

01. ______________________________

______________________________

02. ______________________________

______________________________

03. ______________________________

______________________________

## RELAPSE ______________________________

*(Returning to the place you swore you would never go again. Coping with life on your terms. You sitting in the driver's seat instead of God.)* Giving up and giving in; out of control; lost in your addiction; lying to yourself and others; feeling you just can't manage without your coping behaviors, at least for now. The result is the reinforcement of shame, guilt and condemnation; and feelings of abandonment and being alone.

01. ______________________________

______________________________

02. ______________________________

______________________________

03. ______________________________

______________________________

# Commitment To Change

Complete the Commitment to Change prior to your next group meeting.

Keep in mind, your Commitment to Change is often directly connected to the lowest level reached on the FASTER Scale. Healing happens best when we are fully aware of the challenges we face and take proactive steps to create change.

## LET'S PLAN FOR NEXT WEEK

Commitment to change: what area do you need to change or what challenge are you facing this week?

- Double bind: what will it cost you if you change? If you don't change?
- How does this potential for change make you feel?
- What is your plan to maintain restoration regarding these changes?

Who will you share your commitment with this week?

What are the details of your accountability? What questions should they ask you?

BE PREPARED TO SHARE YOUR ANSWERS IN THIS CHAPTER WITH THE GUYS IN YOUR GROUP.

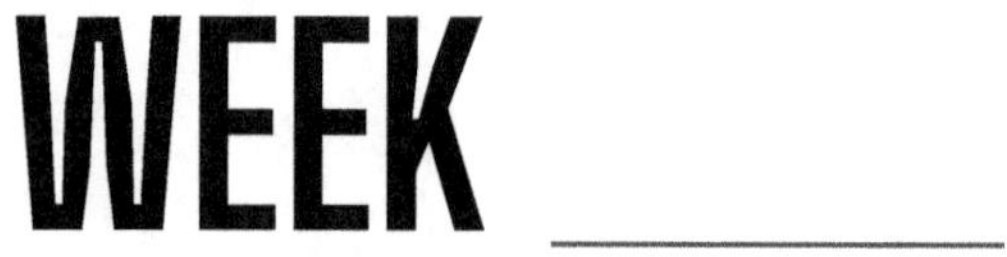

# WEEK ______

## Group Check-In

Complete the Group Check-In 24 hours before group.

### HOW DID YOU DO LAST WEEK?

01. How did you do on your Commitment to Change? ______

02. Did you lie directly or indirectly to anyone? ______

03. What did you do to improve significant relationships with your wife, family, or friends? ______

### WHERE ARE YOU RIGHT NOW?

04. What is the lowest level you identify with on the FASTER Scale? ______

# FASTER Scale

Circle the behaviors on the FASTER Scale that you identify with in each section.
Identify the most powerful behavior in each section and write it next to the corresponding heading.
Answer the following three questions based on your most powerful or frequent behavior.

01. How does it affect me? How do I feel in the moment?
02. How does it affect the important people in my life?
03. Why do I do this? What is the benefit for me?

## RESTORATION ______________________________

*(Accepting life on God's terms, with trust, grace, mercy, vulnerability and gratitude.)* No current secrets; working to resolve problems; identifying fears and feelings; keeping commitments to meetings, prayer, family, church, people, goals, and self; being open and honest, making eye contact; increasing in relationships with God and others; true accountability.

01. ______________________________
02. ______________________________
03. ______________________________

## FORGETTING PRIORITIES ______________________________

*(Start believing the present circumstances and moving away from trusting God. Denial; flight; a change in what's important; how you spend your time, energy, and thoughts.)* Secrets; less time/energy for God, meetings, church; avoiding support and accountability people; superficial conversations; sarcasm; isolating; changes in goals; obsessed with relationships; breaking promises and commitments; neglecting family; preoccupation with material things, TV, computers, entertainment; procrastination; lying; overconfidence; bored; hiding money; image management; seeking to control situations and other people.

01. ______________________________
______________________________
02. ______________________________
______________________________
03. ______________________________
______________________________

## ANXIETY

*(Consumed by negative thoughts and undefined fear; getting energy from emotions.)* Worry, using profanity, being fearful; being resentful; replaying old, negative thoughts; perfectionism; judging other's motives; making goals and lists that you can't complete; mind reading; fantasy, codependent, rescuing; sleep problems, trouble concentrating, seeking/creating drama; gossip; using over-the-counter medication for pain, sleep or weight control; flirting.

01. ______________________________

02. ______________________________

03. ______________________________

## SPEEDING UP

*(Trying to outrun the anxiety which is usually the first sign of depression.)* Super busy and always in a hurry (finding good reason to justify the work); workaholic; can't relax; avoiding slowing down; feeling driven; can't turn off thoughts; skipping meals; binge eating (usually at night); overspending; can't identify own feelings/needs; repetitive negative thoughts; irritable; dramatic mood swings; too much caffeine; over exercising; nervousness; difficulty being alone and/or with people; difficulty listening to others; making excuses for having to "do it all."

01. ______________________________

02. ______________________________

03. ______________________________

## TICKED OFF

*(Getting adrenaline high on anger and aggression.)* Procrastination causing crisis in money, work, and relationships; increased sarcasm; black and white (all or nothing) thinking; feeling alone; nobody understands; overreacting, road rage; constant resentments; pushing others away; increasing isolation; blaming; arguing; irrational thinking; can't take criticism; defensive; people avoiding you; needing to be right; digestive problems; headaches; obsessive (stuck) thoughts; can't forgive; feeling superior; using intimidation.

01. ____________________________________________

____________________________________________

02. ____________________________________________

____________________________________________

03. ____________________________________________

____________________________________________

## EXHAUSTED ____________________________________________

*(Loss of physical and emotional energy; coming off the adrenaline high, and the onset of depression.)* Depressed; panicked; confused; hopelessness; sleeping too much or too little; can't cope; overwhelmed; crying for "no reason"; can't think; forgetful; pessimistic; helpless; tired; numb; wanting to run; constant cravings for old coping behaviors; thinking of using sex, drugs, or alcohol; seeking old unhealthy people and places; really isolating; people angry with you; self abuse; suicidal thoughts; spontaneous crying; no goals; survival mode; not returning phone calls; missing work; irritability; no appetite.

01. ____________________________________________

____________________________________________

02. ____________________________________________

____________________________________________

03. ____________________________________________

____________________________________________

## RELAPSE ____________________________________________

*(Returning to the place you swore you would never go again. Coping with life on your terms. You sitting in the driver's seat instead of God.)* Giving up and giving in; out of control; lost in your addiction; lying to yourself and others; feeling you just can't manage without your coping behaviors, at least for now. The result is the reinforcement of shame, guilt and condemnation; and feelings of abandonment and being alone.

01. ____________________________________________

____________________________________________

02. ____________________________________________

____________________________________________

03. ____________________________________________

____________________________________________

# Commitment To Change

Complete the Commitment to Change prior to your next group meeting.

Keep in mind, your Commitment to Change is often directly connected to the lowest level reached on the FASTER Scale. Healing happens best when we are fully aware of the challenges we face and take proactive steps to create change.

## LET'S PLAN FOR NEXT WEEK

### Commitment to change: what area do you need to change or what challenge are you facing this week?

- Double bind: what will it cost you if you change? If you don't change?
- How does this potential for change make you feel?
- What is your plan to maintain restoration regarding these changes?

### Who will you share your commitment with this week?

### What are the details of your accountability? What questions should they ask you?

**BE PREPARED TO SHARE YOUR ANSWERS IN THIS CHAPTER WITH THE GUYS IN YOUR GROUP.**

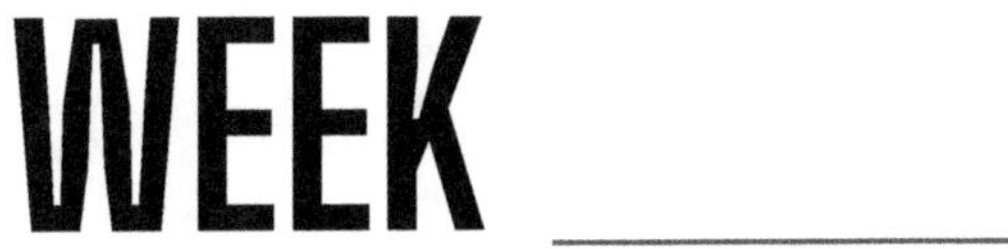

# WEEK ______

## Group Check-In

Complete the Group Check-In 24 hours before group.

### HOW DID YOU DO LAST WEEK?

01. How did you do on your Commitment to Change? ______

02. Did you lie directly or indirectly to anyone? ______

03. What did you do to improve significant relationships with your wife, family, or friends? ______

### WHERE ARE YOU RIGHT NOW?

04. What is the lowest level you identify with on the FASTER Scale? ______

# FASTER Scale

Circle the behaviors on the FASTER Scale that you identify with in each section.
Identify the most powerful behavior in each section and write it next to the corresponding heading.
Answer the following three questions based on your most powerful or frequent behavior.

01. How does it affect me? How do I feel in the moment?
02. How does it affect the important people in my life?
03. Why do I do this? What is the benefit for me?

## RESTORATION ______________________________

*(Accepting life on God's terms, with trust, grace, mercy, vulnerability and gratitude.)* No current secrets; working to resolve problems; identifying fears and feelings; keeping commitments to meetings, prayer, family, church, people, goals, and self; being open and honest, making eye contact; increasing in relationships with God and others; true accountability.

01. ______________________________
02. ______________________________
03. ______________________________

## FORGETTING PRIORITIES ______________________________

*(Start believing the present circumstances and moving away from trusting God. Denial; flight; a change in what's important; how you spend your time, energy, and thoughts.)* Secrets; less time/energy for God, meetings, church; avoiding support and accountability people; superficial conversations; sarcasm; isolating; changes in goals; obsessed with relationships; breaking promises and commitments; neglecting family; preoccupation with material things, TV, computers, entertainment; procrastination; lying; overconfidence; bored; hiding money; image management; seeking to control situations and other people.

01. ______________________________
______________________________
02. ______________________________
______________________________
03. ______________________________
______________________________

## ANXIETY

*(Consumed by negative thoughts and undefined fear; getting energy from emotions.)* Worry, using profanity, being fearful; being resentful; replaying old, negative thoughts; perfectionism; judging other's motives; making goals and lists that you can't complete; mind reading; fantasy, codependent, rescuing; sleep problems, trouble concentrating, seeking/creating drama; gossip; using over-the-counter medication for pain, sleep or weight control; flirting.

01. ______________________________

02. ______________________________

03. ______________________________

## SPEEDING UP

*(Trying to outrun the anxiety which is usually the first sign of depression.)* Super busy and always in a hurry (finding good reason to justify the work); workaholic; can't relax; avoiding slowing down; feeling driven; can't turn off thoughts; skipping meals; binge eating (usually at night); overspending; can't identify own feelings/needs; repetitive negative thoughts; irritable; dramatic mood swings; too much caffeine; over exercising; nervousness; difficulty being alone and/or with people; difficulty listening to others; making excuses for having to "do it all."

01. ______________________________

02. ______________________________

03. ______________________________

## TICKED OFF

*(Getting adrenaline high on anger and aggression.)* Procrastination causing crisis in money, work, and relationships; increased sarcasm; black and white (all or nothing) thinking; feeling alone; nobody understands; overreacting, road rage; constant resentments; pushing others away; increasing isolation; blaming; arguing; irrational thinking; can't take criticism; defensive; people avoiding you; needing to be right; digestive problems; headaches; obsessive (stuck) thoughts; can't forgive; feeling superior; using intimidation.

01. ______________________________________________

______________________________________________

02. ______________________________________________

______________________________________________

03. ______________________________________________

______________________________________________

## EXHAUSTED

*(Loss of physical and emotional energy; coming off the adrenaline high, and the onset of depression.)* Depressed; panicked; confused; hopelessness; sleeping too much or too little; can't cope; overwhelmed; crying for "no reason"; can't think; forgetful; pessimistic; helpless; tired; numb; wanting to run; constant cravings for old coping behaviors; thinking of using sex, drugs, or alcohol; seeking old unhealthy people and places; really isolating; people angry with you; self abuse; suicidal thoughts; spontaneous crying; no goals; survival mode; not returning phone calls; missing work; irritability; no appetite.

01. ______________________________________________

______________________________________________

02. ______________________________________________

______________________________________________

03. ______________________________________________

______________________________________________

## RELAPSE

*(Returning to the place you swore you would never go again. Coping with life on your terms. You sitting in the driver's seat instead of God.)* Giving up and giving in; out of control; lost in your addiction; lying to yourself and others; feeling you just can't manage without your coping behaviors, at least for now. The result is the reinforcement of shame, guilt and condemnation; and feelings of abandonment and being alone.

01. ______________________________________________

______________________________________________

02. ______________________________________________

______________________________________________

03. ______________________________________________

______________________________________________

# Commitment To Change

Complete the Commitment to Change prior to your next group meeting.

Keep in mind, your Commitment to Change is often directly connected to the lowest level reached on the FASTER Scale. Healing happens best when we are fully aware of the challenges we face and take proactive steps to create change.

## LET'S PLAN FOR NEXT WEEK

Commitment to change: what area do you need to change or what challenge are you facing this week?

- Double bind: what will it cost you if you change? If you don't change?
- How does this potential for change make you feel?
- What is your plan to maintain restoration regarding these changes?

Who will you share your commitment with this week?

What are the details of your accountability? What questions should they ask you?

BE PREPARED TO SHARE YOUR ANSWERS IN THIS CHAPTER WITH THE GUYS IN YOUR GROUP.

www.ingramcontent.com/pod-product-compliance
Lightning Source LLC
LaVergne TN
LVHW080333110826
845155LV00027B/234

*9781943291229*